Chi Kung

"Taoist Secrets of Fitness and Longevity"

BY

WEN MEI YU

up

Disclaimer:

Although both Unique Publications and the author(s) of this martial book have taken great care to ensure the authenticity of the information and techniques contained herein, we are not responsible, in whole or part, for any injury which may occur to the reader or readers by reading and/or following the instruction in this publication. We also do not guarantee that the techniques and illustrations described in this book will be safe and effective in a self-defense training or situation. It is understood that there exist a potential for injury when using or demonstrating the techniques herein described. It is essential that before following any of the activities, physical or otherwise, herein described, the reader or readers first should consult his or her physician for advise on whether practicing or using the techniques described in this publication could cause injury physical or otherwise. Since the physical activities described herein could be too sophisticated in nature for the reader or readers, it is essential a physician be consulted. Also federal, state or local laws may prohibit the use or possession of weapons described herein. A thorough examination must be made of the federal, state and local laws before the rader or readers attempts to use these weapons in a self-defense situation or otherwise. Neiother unique Publications nor the autnor(s) of this martial arts book guarantees the legality or the appropriateness of the techniques or weapons herein contained.

Library of Congress Catalog No. - 97-62166
ISBN: 0-86568-165-1

Published by Unique Publications

Printed in the United States of America

up UNIQUE PUBLICATIONS
4201 Vanowen Place, Burbank, CA 91505

TABLE OF CONTENTS

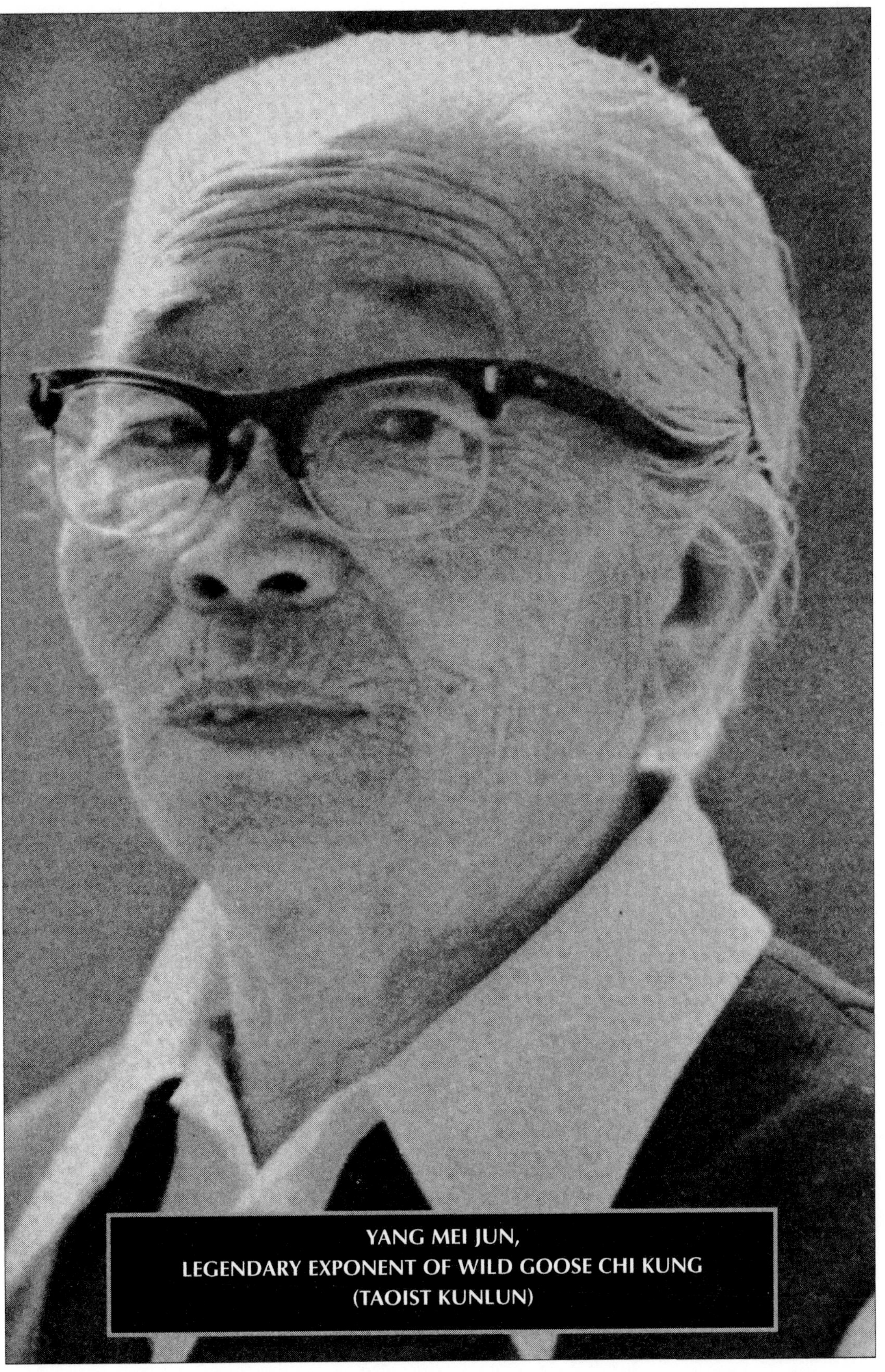

YANG MEI JUN,
LEGENDARY EXPONENT OF WILD GOOSE CHI KUNG
(TAOIST KUNLUN)

AUTHORS' NOTE

When English spellings are used for Chinese words, "Q" will be used to describe the "Ch" sound, and "G" for the "G" sound. Only in the words Chi, Kung, or Chi Kung will this rule be altered. In this case, the "Ch" spelling will be used to describe the "Ch" sound, and the "K" spelling used to described the "G" sound. Otherwise we hope this book is practical and useful to you, regardless of your knowledge and love for the art of Chi Kung.

CHAPTER ONE:

CHI KUNG'S ORIGINS

Chi Kung (or, Qigong) is the ancient Chinese art of strengthening health to prevent and treat diseases and prolong life. Chi translates to Air and Energy, and Kung refers to hard work, talent, or the exercise associated with hard work and the display of talent. Chi Kung, translates meaning "Breathing Exercise."

Chi Kung practitioners often concern themselves with the development, assimilation and storage of Chi (Vital Energy). The practitioner often feels sensations when contacting energy, and very often these sensations manifest in the form of warmth and tingling. Some practitioners compare these sensations of energy to static electricity or particle stream.

Chi Kung practice usually involves the attainment of skills, that allow the practitioner to gather, dispel, direct, and store Chi (Vital Energy). Therefore the work, or practice of Chi Kung helps to develop the practitioner's Kung (Skill or talent), and the practitioner's health and strength generally improves with the amount of quality work in which the practitioner engages.

Quality of work is important to consider. In the ancient philosophical aspects of training, which is still carried on today, there is a belief in developing a strong foundation from the ground up when practicing or learning anything; and Chi Kung is no exception. Correct foot work, hand methods, and techniques are considered essential for deeper understanding, and beneficial, long term practice.

Granted people have a variety of body shapes, energies, and belief systems. Yet appropriate body mechanics enables the practitioner to apply Physical Science, and combine movements which encourage the flow of energy with the Science of Acu-Meridian therapy which is utilized in traditional Chinese massage and acupuncture. In fact, Chi Kung itself is an integral part of ancient Chinese medicine.

THE FIVE BRANCHES

Chi Kung is generally divided into five branches which are as follows: Taoist, Confucian, Buddhist, Medical, and Martial. Within these five branches are various sects, schools, and sub groupings. Also, within each of the sects, schools, or sub groupings are a variety of differences; as well as, similarities.

The Taoist branch first considers strengthening the body and mind. Contrary to some viewpoints, the "Tao" is not achieved by "doing nothing." While it's true nature is at the utmost concern to achieve the higher levels of practice and understanding, initially that's not the case.

It is only after the techniques become second nature, and the mind and body developed and brought into harmony, that the emphasis shifts to following or "flowing" with nature, or utilizing the natural laws of motion. Furthermore, at this stage of practice, emphasis is placed on the "emptying of the mind." Moreover, that the mind follow the movement that is following the natural laws of motion. In this way the outcome or effect cannot be predetermined. Only the initial movement that sets the whole system into motion is known. Even the end result can be known, but the path is what remains the mystery.

This doesn't mean that a predetermined form is not utilized. Rather, that the practitioner allows natural forces of motion such as gravity, centrifugal force, and momentum to determine the twists, turns, squats, steps, etc. to accomplish the elements of a form.

In the Confucian branch the emphasis is strongly on self cultivation through sincerity, and regulating the mind and thoughts. During the Spring and Autumn and Warring States Period (770-221 B.C.), the Confucians researched and developed Chi Kung practice. It is their belief that semen, internal energy, and the mind are regarded as three treasures that a person should protect and master control over. Never allowing one's heart to get carried away by what one sees, or otherwise senses. The practice consists of encouraging the practitioner to reach a state of rest, calm, and quiet in all things.

In the Buddhist branch, the mind remains central in all practices. Meditation is the ultimate goal of the mind's work. The body is seen as secondary to the mind, and serves as a vehicle to develop, progress, and achieve enlightenment. Buddhist forms often combine external, as well as internal methods. The emphasis is on a technique known as a pumping of the Chi, which involves combining the full extent of force changing to a full extent of relaxation. Changing both gradually, as well as suddenly. Another example, is when water is traveling through a garden hose, and the hose is pinched or stepped on, the water stops flowing completely through. Then when you suddenly let go or take the foot off, the water suddenly flows more from the sudden release of built up pressure. This

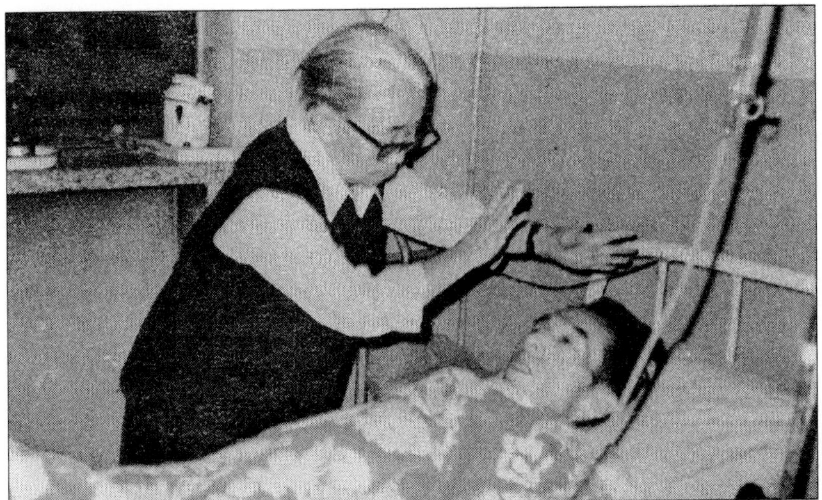

Yang Mei Jun, legendary exponent of the Wild Goose Chi Kung School, administers the Directed Healing method to a patient.

method is applied at times in Taoist systems, and in contemporary developments of Chi Kung. However, the traditional Buddhist technique trains the mind in form's practice to go to the fullest extent of force, and to the fullest extent of relaxation.

In the Medical branch, the primary purpose is to treat diseases. However optimum results are often achieved in prevention. Medical Chi Kung often involves three areas: Directed Healing, Self Controlled Therapy, and Hands On Therapy. Directed Healing can at first appear fake to many Westerners. Even within the borders of China there exists some skepticism despite a wide array of scientific research. The Directed Healing Method calls for the advanced practitioner or physician to direct their energy into specific points or channels on the patient's body in order that various circulations can be encouraged for the purpose of dispelling bad Chi, and encouraging circulation for developing or strengthening the system.

It's important for the transmitter to be knowledgeable and possess good qualifications and skills. Otherwise without proper training and knowledge, the patient's problem(s) could magnify and become worse, instead of better. It also helps if the patient can trust and believe in the transmission administered by the physician. Thereby involving the patient in the healing process by inciting them to become an active participant.

Self Controlled Therapy calls on the patient to practice certain movements or techniques aimed at curing or preventing sickness. This is the most popular among patients who have prolonged their life or overcome their disease or sickness. Giving the patient a form that they can do, gives them a sense of accomplishment when they finish a certain form's requirements. However, this doesn't have to be a one size fits all approach. Depending upon the patient's ability or condition, the form may have to be designed or tailored to be effective and fit the patient's particular needs.

Hands On Healing usually refers to Massage such as: Tui Na or Acupressure, which are an integral part of Traditional Chinese Medicine. Thereby the physician or therapist places their hands or fingers on certain points, muscle groups, joints, etc. Softening these areas and connective tissue, in order that the Chi may begin to flow.

Martial Chi Kung refers to the Martial Arts both external and internal. Some internal martial artists believe that they are privy to the idea of Chi Kung and the development of Chi. While it is true that the slower, deliberate, relaxed training methods (often associated with internal arts systems) emphasizes Chi Kung methods, and the development of Chi, it is widely accepted that the internal arts developed from the external arts.

Some external styles include their own internal sets or teach internal methods from the beginning. However, beginners in the external arts often don't understand the internal aspects of their art until they persevere over a long period of time in arduous practice. Ironically, the same could be said for internal practitioners as well.

THE ANCIENT METHOD OF DAOYIN

According to Guo Moruo, a late well known historian and former President of the Chinese Academy of Sciences, there were records of a breathing exercise in the "jin wen" (or, Writings on Bronzes) of the Zhou Dynasty (1100-221 B.C.).

During the Spring and Autumn and the Warring States Periods (770-221 B.C.) the Confucians investigated the theories of Chi Kung. In the Book of Changes by Confucius, semen, internal energy, and the mind were regarded as three treasures a person should preserve and master control over.

Also at this time, the ancient exercise of Daoyin (A breathing, fitness exercise) flourished. In the earliest extant medical classic written during this period, Huang Di Neijing (The Yellow Emperor's Manual of Internal Medicine) a breathing exercise is described as follows:

"A person must breathe the essence of life, regulate their respiration to safeguard their spirit, and keep the muscles relaxed."

Another part suggests to do the following for kidney trouble:

"Stand with the face turned to the south in the early morning and breathe in seven times without a thought and a clear mind."

On a cultural relic of the Warring States period, the following words are engraved:

"Inhale deeply, and sink the energy of the air to the Lower Dantian (An acu-meridian area located just below the navel, and encompassing the lower abdomen). Retain the breath, and gradually exhale as if blowing on a flute. Allowing the energy to go up through the top of your head. In this way you will train your Yang (or, masculine) energy to go up, and your Yin (or, feminine) energy to go down."

The Baihui point located at the top of your head is where all the body's Yang channels collect. The Huiyin located between the sexual organs (scrotum or vagina) and anus is where all the body's Yin channels collect. Daoyin's practice involves a separating of the energies through these two points, thereby the body's energies would flow correctly and balance achieved. It was believed during the Warring States Period, when Daoyin was known to have been practiced that death could come to those who's energy flowed incorrectly, and imbalances occurred.

Daoyin can be better understood by breaking the word down into two parts, "Dao" and "Yin" as follows:

> "Dao" refers to the cerebral cortex, and that it be placed in a state of alert tranquility. It is in this calm, yet alert state that the Chi (Vital Energy) can flow. The blood flow is healthy, uninterrupted, and sensed. Pulsations can be felt at various points throughout the internal and external aspects of the body. Aside from the more readily identified pulsations of the neck and wrist.
>
> "Yin" refers to movement, and to allow movements to occur which encourage the Vital Energy to flow with great ease, and to encourage the oxygen flow to be fresh and precise. As long as the tranquil, yet alert state is encouraged, the mind and body can relax. As long as the movements incorporated are smooth and encourage the energy to flow through specific channels, the Chi flow will usually be strong and useful.

Chi Kung practice becomes even more effective when the hands are employed to radiate the Chi. The hands, because of their natural ability to move and contact Chi from any direction whether up, down, behind, or front are great conductors of energy. Just slowly moving the hands in front of each other, or together and apart from each other, energy can be sensed in the hands without a great degree of difficulty. Ancient research into the incorporation of the hands as conductors of energy very likely led to the development of more sophisticated schools of Chi Kung some time around 208 A.D.

FROM HUA TUO'S DISCOVERIES TO DAO AN

A famous promoter of Daoyin was Hua Tuo a famous Physician in China during the Han Dynasty (206 BC-220 AD). Not much is known of Hua Tuo's practices, other than he was primarily concerned with prevention of disease.

As the story goes, Hua Tuo became frustrated with constantly receiving patients often suffering from diseases or disorders very often in the terminal stages. Hua Tuo became sure the only way to cure disease was to avoid it, or prevent it, to begin with.

Through a series of experiments, Hua Tuo promoted a set of exercises handed down to him through ancient times known as Daoyin. Exactly how the exercises worked or what order they were arranged in is unknown. However, there is research that suggests that Hua Tuo may have revised the popular exercise "Six Animal Game", and actually compiled the famous "Five Animal Game" (or, Wuqinxi) which imitates the postures and behavior of the tiger seizing, the deer stretching, the bear crawling, the monkey jumping, and the bird flying. Some accounts mark him as the creator of Five Animal Game.

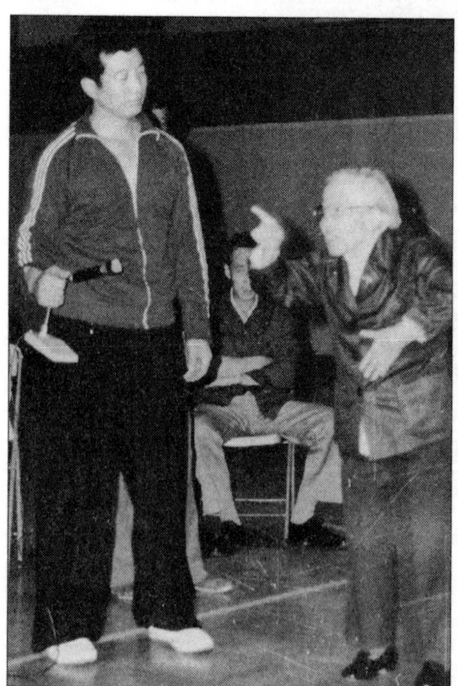

Yang Mei Jun lectures in Shanghai on the benefits of Chi Kung practice.

Among the medical books discovered in 1973 from Tomb No. III of the Han Dynasty at Ma Wang Dui, Changsha, China, there are two articles which describe the uses of Daoyin. Accompanying the two articles are more than forty illustrations of Daoyin. Astonishingly, the drawings are in good shape and well preserved.

Mystery surrounds the death of Hua Tuo, who is said to have looked like a young man into his old age, and passed on the essence of his research and teachings to his disciples secretly and selectively. One thing for sure, most accounts recognize Hua Tuo as an early Chi Kung pioneer, who at any rate laid a foundation for the continuation and development of Chi Kung that is practiced and developed upon until this day.

It was also at this time that three different schools of Chi Kung would develop: Kunlun, Kong Tong, and Shaolin. The Wild Goose Chi Kung would later develop in the Taoist Kunlun school in

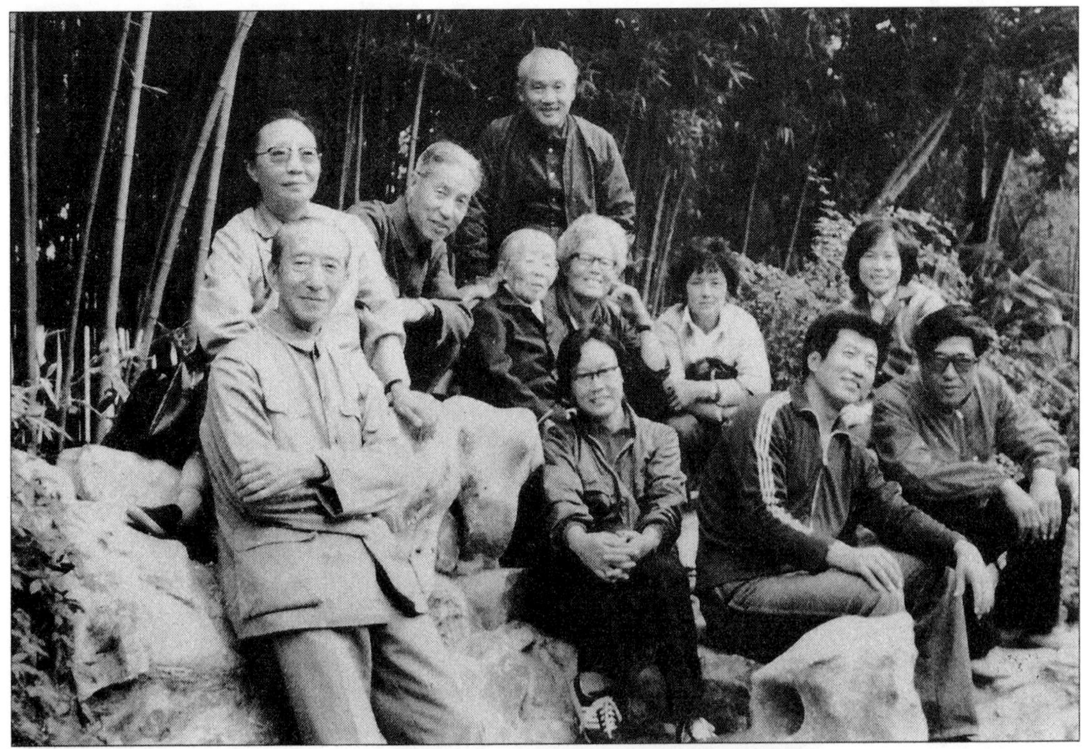

Yang Mei Jun with students taking a break after an intense practice session. Below Yang Mei Jun in the foreground is Wen Mei Yu.

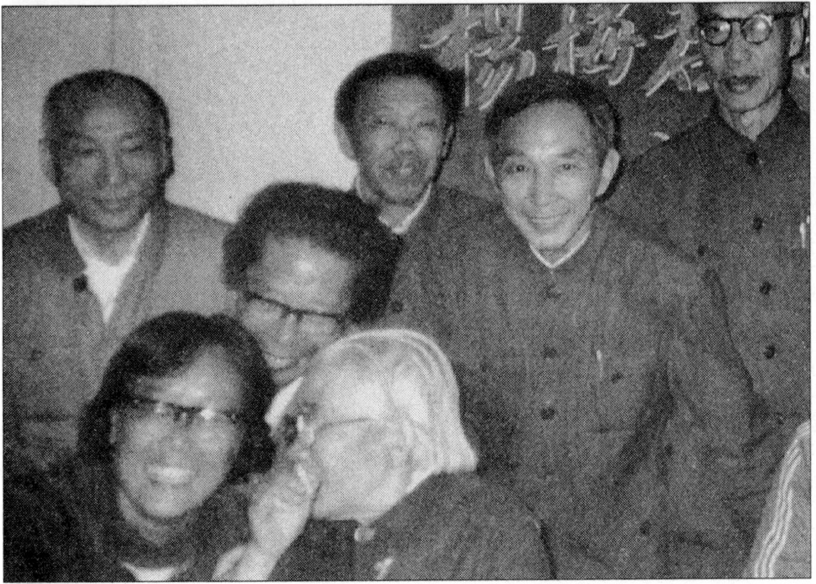

Yang Mei Jun and Wen Mei Yu sharing a personal moment together.

Sichuan during the Jin Dynasty.

From the Han Dynasty to the Tang Dynasty, Chi Kung and related methods continued to be used in medical treatment. Chao Yuan fang, a Chi Kung practitioner and physician in the Sui Dynasty (581-618) pointed out that when a person had fully

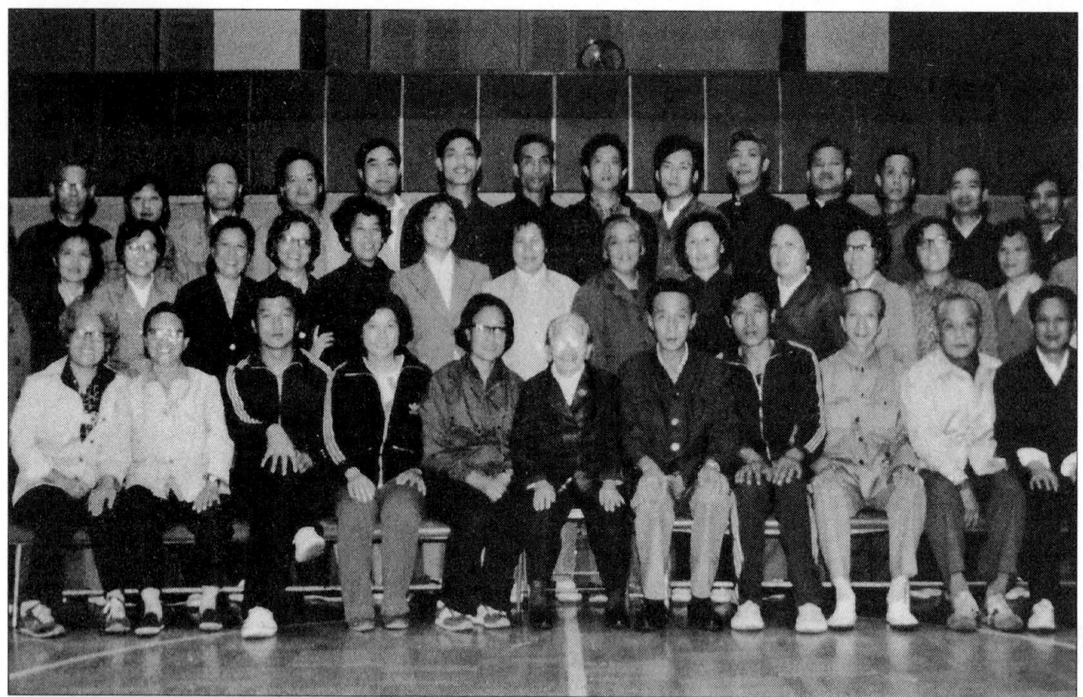

Wild Goose Chi Kung Graduating Class in Shanghai: Sixth from right is Yang Mei Jun, and seventh from right is Wen Mei Yu.

acquired the knowledge of Chi Kung, that they could emit from their palm a type of vital energy or chi to cure diseases for others.

Sun Simao (581-682) was also a famous physician who authored a book known as One Thousand Prescriptions. In it he clarified and detailed the theory and practice of Daoyin.

Chi Kung would survive through the Song and Qing Dynasties (960-1911). Often developed among religious sects and martial artists for spiritual development , power, and energy, and serving as vehicles for enlightenment through arduous practice. Often these methods were kept secret for fear of placing power in the hands of evil doers or enemies.

Dayan, or Wild Goose, Chi Kung developed out of the Taoist Kunlun School, which developed in Sichuan province during the Jin dynasty. The most prolific teacher at that time was Dao An, believed to be an early ancestor of Dayan (or, Wild Goose) Chi Kung.

From the Jin dynasty to the Chen dynasty, the system was very secretive, and only a few were recognized to continue teaching and passing it on.

After Dao An's death, Dayan (or, Wild Goose) Chi Kung developed in the northern part of China. Wan Yi, an elder monk from Wu Tai mountain, would record in detail the history and substance of the Wild Goose Chi Kung system for many generations to come. In his records it was also noted that traditionally unless a person had practiced for some time and their age was over 70 years, the person was not fit to teach the system.

Yang Mei Jun, considered one of the most prolific teachers of Wild Goose Chi Kung in modern times, began her training in the Taoist Kunlun School began at age 13 under her grandfather, Yang De Shan (who at the time was 73 years old).

It is said that while some Masters ran indoors for warmth during the icy winters in Beijing, Yang Mei Jun is said to have continued her practice outdoors, wearing only thin clothing. On the winter evenings after intense practice, Yang Mei Jun would lay down on a cold park bench and circulate her Chi. Storing it in her Lower Dantian (An acu-meridian area located below the navel, and encompassing the lower abdomen.) to create a fire to warm her body. In this way she knew her practice of circulating Chi was really correct.

Yang Mei Jun's life changed dramatically during the Japanese occupation of China in the 1940's. Her father was a rickshaw driver who would carry Japanese drivers from place to place.

One night, Yang Mei Jun's father picked up a drunken Japanese soldier who stabbed him in the back with a bayonet while prodding him to go faster.

Yang Mei Jun was left alone, and had to rely on neighbors to bury her father; she was poor and unable to do so herself. Yang Mei Jun would then assume the role of a man, to survive in a cruel world.

Masquerading as a man, she worked side by side with men illegally selling salt which was forbidden by the Japanese during the occupation. It was at this time she met her husband, and together they joined guerrilla forces in the countryside to fight the Japanese.

Captured at one point, she and five others were buried alive to die a torturous death. Under the ground, Yang Mei Jun remained calm, circulating her Chi, and practicing internal breathing. Sensing the soldier's departure, she dug her way out, and saved others as well from emanate death.

Her persistence in practice of Wild Goose Chi Kung continued through other difficult times. It is in times of adversity, that Yang Mei Jun discovered the reality of Chi Kung. It was also during these times that her Chi Kung level developed to new heights. None would be more challenging than her persecution during the Cultural Revolution in China (1966-1974).

Like many other great martial artists, she was made to suffer for her practices. The Red Guard made her sit for hours in a public place to suffer public embarrassment and scrutiny. She practiced remaining calm and circulating her Chi. When forced to stand, she continued to practice by having her ten toes grip the ground, clearing her mind, maintaining a pure heart, and projecting a peaceful spirit.

In 1978, Yang Mei Jun's husband passed on. Also at that time China began to open up more politically. Realizing her responsibility to pass on Wild Goose Chi Kung (as her age was over 70 years old), Yang Mei Jun began offering instruction in Wild Goose Chi Kung to the public. Her first classes were held at Xuan Wu Park in Beijing.

CHAPTER TWO:

CHANNELS, MERIDIANS, POINTS AND THEORY: CHI KUNG'S MAP OF HEALTH AND CONSCIOUSNESS

The human body has a special system or map that connects the exterior with the interior, as well as the upper and the lower portions of the body. The channels connect the solid and hollow internal organs of the body with sensitive areas on the body known as "points." The sensitive points are often connected to the channels or meridians. The channels are not to be confused with blood vessels or nerves.

The channels are routes, the meridians are major routes, and the points are special contact or emission places located mostly on channels or meridians. Like a bus system of a major city, the Chi is intended to flow ideally like the buses uninhibited by traffic. However, when there is a jam or an accident directly or indirectly involving a bus on a major or minor street or intersection, there is a delay or stoppage in traffic.

Similarly, when the Chi stops flowing through the channels (minor routes) or meridians (major routes), or at a specific point, a pain or problem may rise. Chi Kung Practitioners often refer to the body's Chi stopped or being "stuck" at a particular point, or along a channel or meridian when a physical problem develops. An accident of energies can occur from stress, over inducement of pollution, bad food, and other related problems associated with everyday living.

Incorrect Chi Kung practice can cause problems as well. Like other forms of exercise, incorrect Chi Kung practice can cause problems that can sometimes surpass problems such as hyperextension, often associated with excessive physical stress. Because Chi Kung deals with internal energy, incorrect use or improper application of energy, can cause an accident to occur on the channels.

Chi Kung practice can vary in style and system, and what route the Chi takes varies from style to style or system to system as well. That's why it's important to practice one type of Chi Kung at a time.

For the beginner, they should emphasize the practice of one particular type of Chi Kung for at least a month or more before beginning practice of another type of Chi Kung (even within the same branch or sect). For the advanced practitioner who may have studied various types of Chi Kung over a period of years, it is not harmful to practice one type of Chi Kung in the morning and another type in the evening. However, some practitioners wait a twenty four period before adopting a different style or method, to allow the Chi to work it's entire course in relationship to time. Every two hours of the day correlates to the most optimal time to practice to effect one of the twelve channels of the body (See The "Chi" Clock, Chapter 3).

As we examine the twelve channels, eight meridians, and basic points emphasized in Wild Goose Chi Kung understand that there exists a variety of opinions that vary slightly throughout the world concerning the precise branches, location, and path of the channels, meridians, and points. We are all different and naturally the precise location of points, paths and branches of channels and meridians will vary from person to person. Acu-Meridian theory is always being argued, examined, researched, tested, and updated like any other valid Science. Hopefully the information contained herein will provide the reader with a basic or interesting overview that will create opinions, questions, and most of all encourage more personal interest and research.

A. THE TWELVE CHANNELS

There are twelve regular channels. The twelve regular channels lead to the solid (or, Yin) and hollow (or, Yang) organs. The channels have two characters, Yin and Yang. Those channels that go along the interior part of the body are called yin channels. The channels that go along the outside part of the body are called yang channels. They are classified as: three yin channels of the hand that lead to solid organs (Lung, Heart, and Pericardium); three yang channels of the hand that lead to hollow organs (Large Intestine, Small Intestine, and Triple Warmer); three yin channels of the foot that lead to solid organs (Spleen, Kidney, and Liver); and three yang channels of the foot that lead to hollow organs (Stomach, Urinary Bladder, and Gall Bladder).

The twelve channels are joined theoretically as follows: The three yin channels of the hand extend from the chest and through the hand to join the three yang channels of the hand. The three yang channels of the hand extend from the hand and through the head to join three yang channels of the foot. The three yang channels of the foot extend from the head and through the foot to join the three yin channels of the foot. Finally, the three yin channels of the foot extend from the foot , through the chest , and join the three yin channels of the hand.

The twelve channels are drawn and described in Figures A1-A12 as:

The Lung Channel of the Hand (Taiyin), and The Large Intestine Channel of the Hand (Yangming); The Stomach Channel of the Foot (Yangming), and The Spleen Channel of the Foot (Taiyin); The Heart Channel of the Hand (Shaoyin), and The Small Intestine of the Hand (Taiyang); The Urinary Bladder Channel of the Foot (Taiyang), and The Kidney Channel of the Foot (Shaoyin); The Pericardium Channel of the Hand (Jueyin), and The Triple Warmer Channel of the Hand (Shaoyang); The Gallbladder Channel of the Foot (Shaoyang), and The Liver Channel of the Foot (Jueyin).

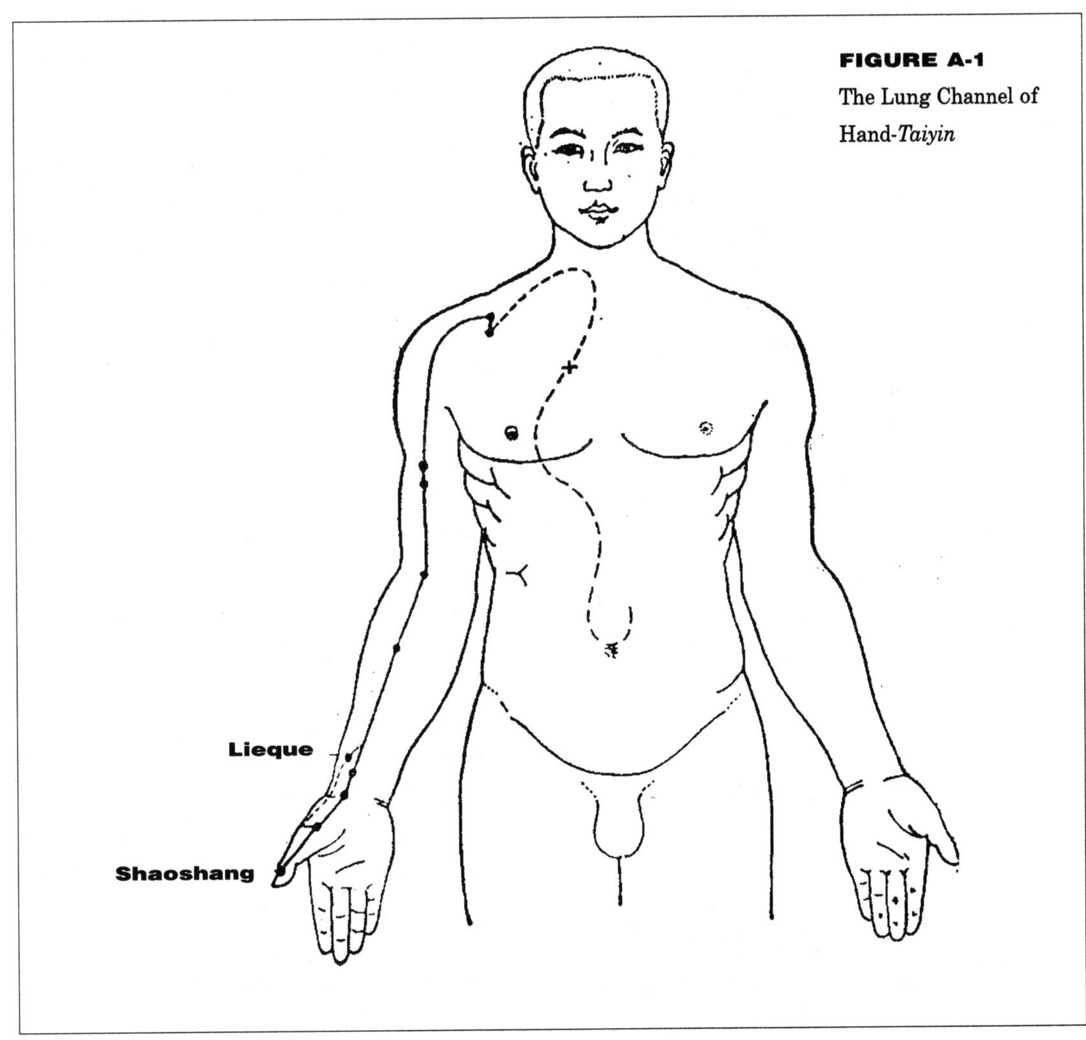

FIGURE A-1

The Lung Channel of Hand-*Taiyin*

1. THE LUNG CHANNEL OF THE HAND (TAIYIN)

The Lung Channel of the Hand (Taiyin) begins internally in the pelvic region and connects with the large intestine. Then goes up to the stomach, and continues up past the diaphragm. Passing through the lung and it proceeds laterally from the trachea (windpipe) to the clavicle, and exits superficially. Descends the middle of the upper arm to the elbow. Continues descending along the forearm dividing at the Lieque point, while continuing it's descent through the front of the radial artery. Then continuing along the back and front boundary of the hand, and stopping on the thumb at the Shaoshang point. A branch runs from the Lieque point along the back of the forefinger to the fingertip, and there connects to the Large Intestine Channel of the Hand (Yangming) at the Shangyang point.

Careful and correct stimulation of this channel may help relieve: Stuffiness in the chest, chest pains, irritability, sweaty

FIGURE A-2
The Large intestine Channel of Hand-*Yangming*

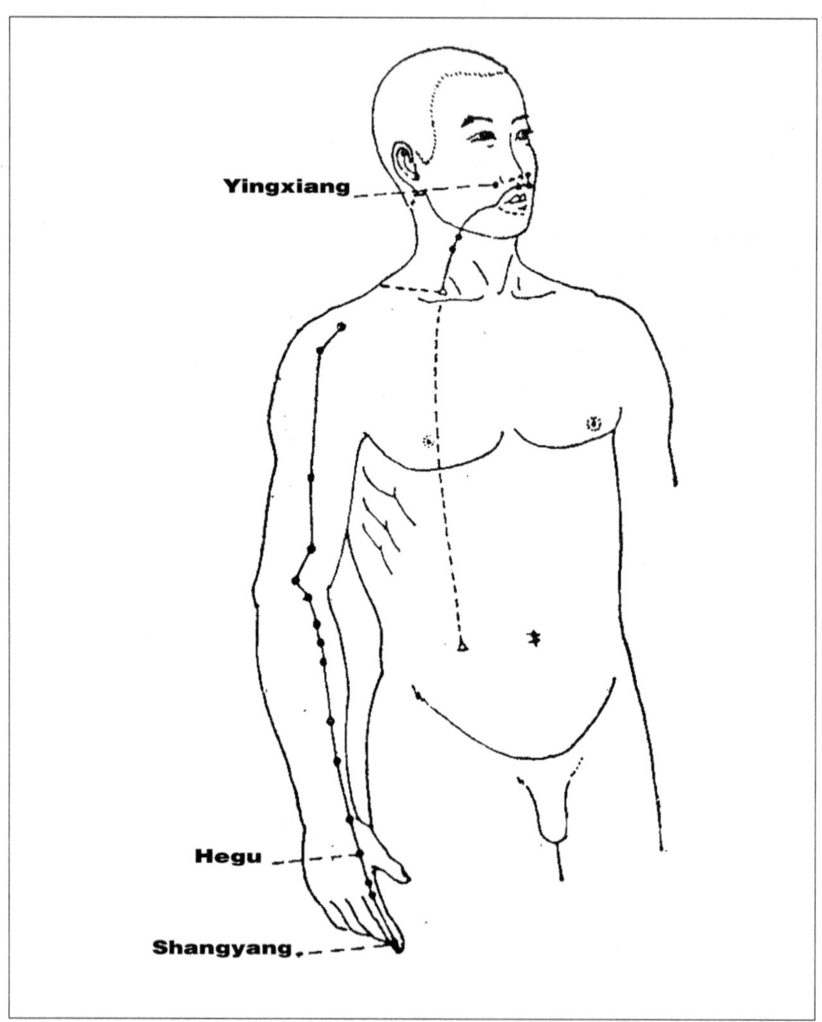

palms, pains in the arms, sore throat, back and shoulder pain, bronchitis, and a recurring cold.

2. THE LARGE INTESTINE CHANNEL OF THE HAND (YANGMING)

The Large Intestine Channel of the Hand (Yangming) begins at the tip of the forefinger at the Shangyang point. Going up along the back and front boundary of the forefinger, and passing through the Hegu point. Continuing up along the side of the forearm, and passing through the side of the crook of the elbow. Continuing up along the side of the arm, the line crosses through the Small Intestine Channel of the Hand (Taiyang). Goes back to above the clavicle, and divides into two branches. The internal branch goes into the chest and connects with the lung, passes through the diaphragm, and descends to the large intestine. Then converging with the Spleen Channel of the Foot (Taiyin). The superficial branch goes up from above the clavicle to the neck, continues up to the lower jaw bone, and connects internally with the lower teeth. Encircling the upper lip and ends at the Yingxiang point near the nose. There linking with the Stomach Channel of the Foot (Yangming).

FIGURE A-3
The Stomach Channel of Foot-*Yangmiong*

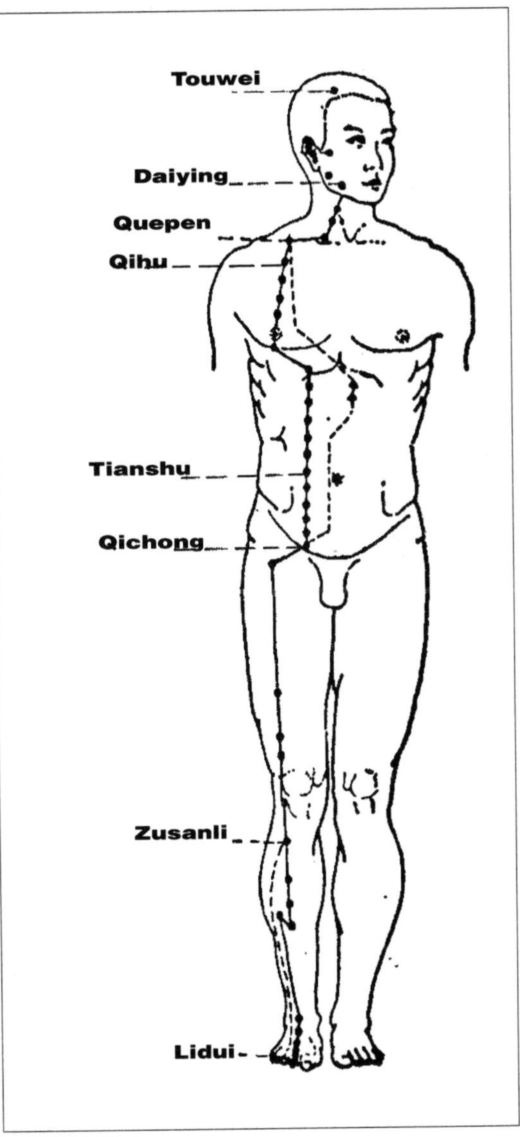

Careful and correct stimulation of this channel may help relieve: Running nose, stuffed nose, epistaxis (nose bleed), sore throat, dryness in the mouth, chronic abdominal pain with diarrhea, habitual constipation, shoulder pain, and early cervical spondylosis (stiffness of a vertebral joint of the spine).

3. THE STOMACH CHANNEL OF THE FOOT (YANGMING)

The Stomach Channel of the Foot (Yangming) begins at the Yingxiang point by the nose and ascends to the upper end of the nose bridge, crossing the Urinary Bladder Channel of the Foot (Taiyang), and descending along the side of the nose. There entering the upper gum, and emerging and curving around the lips. Then running along the back and underside of the saliva glands through the Daiying point. Ascending in front of the ear, and running along the hairline to the forehead to the Touwei point.

A branch from the Daiying point descends along the front of the neck, and winds over to the Quepen point above the clavicle where it splits into two branches.

An internal branch descends from the Quepen point, and goes past the Diaphragm. Passing through the stomach, connecting with the Ren Meridian, and finally connecting with the spleen.

A superficial branch descends from the Quepen point, passing through Qihu, and to the nipple. Runs further down past Tianshu, and reaches the Qichong point.

The internal branch has a branch that goes from the stomach which descends internally to the Qichong point to join up with the superficial branch. Now joined, the channel descends to the knee. Continuing downward along the side of the Tibia (Shin bone), and continuing from and branching at the Zusanli point. Continuing down through the middle part of the foot splitting with one branch ending at the Lidui point on the side of the second toe.

A Tibial (Shin bone) branch descends from the Zusanli point, and terminates at the side of the third toe. A branch sent out from the middle part of the foot reaches the Yinbai point at the middle of the big toe. Thereby connecting with the Spleen Channel of the Foot (Taiyin).

Careful and correct stimulation of this channel may help relieve: Gastrointestinal disorder and disease, and diseases related to the head, face, eye, nose, mouth, teeth, and the anterior aspect of the lower extremity. As well as, continued shivering, repeated yawning, black and dark colorization of the frontal skin. Rapid digestion, uncontrollable hunger, and yellowish urine are possible further indications of a hindered Stomach channel.

FIGURE A-4

The Spleen Channel of Foot-*Taiyin*

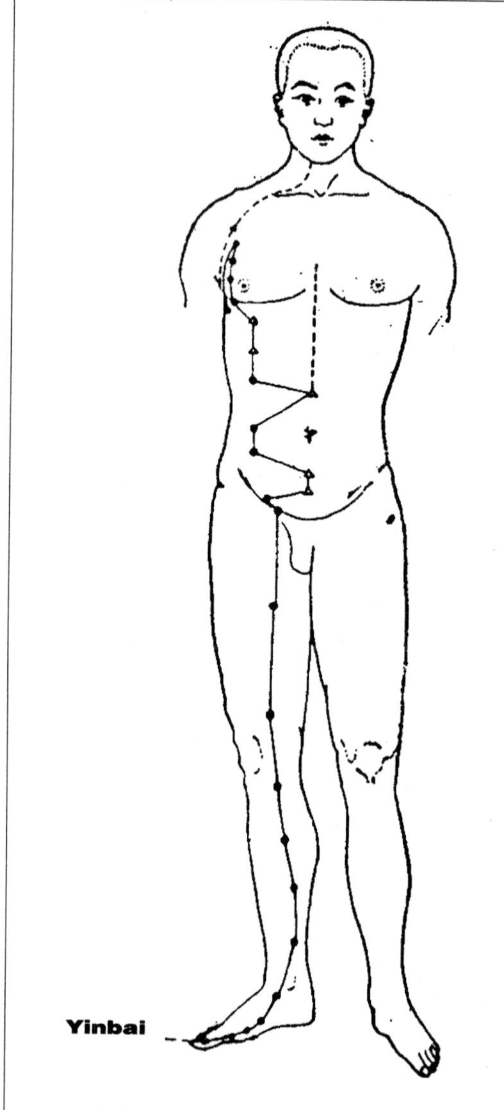

4. THE SPLEEN CHANNEL OF THE FOOT (TAIYIN)

Originating at the middle of the big toe at the Yinbai point, the Spleen Channel of the Foot (Taiyin) ascends along the back and front boundary of the middle of the big toe, and reaching the front of the middle of the ankle. Continuing to travel upwards along the back of the Tibia (Shin bone), and ascending up in front of the Liver Channel of the Foot (Jueyin). Going through the front of the middle of the knee and thigh, and into the abdomen. Then entering the spleen, passing the stomach, and going through the diaphragm. Continuing upwards along the two sides of the throat, reaching the root of the tongue, and spreading over it's lower surface.

The branch of the channel that splits off from the stomach, goes upward through the diaphragm, dispersing into the heart, and connecting with the Heart Channel of the Hand (Shaoyin).

Careful and correct stimulation of this channel may help relieve: Abdominal tension, stiff tongue, indigestion, chronic diarrhea, impotence, involuntary seminal emission, jaundice, stomach ache, vomiting after meals, swelling of the middle portion of the thigh, knee, or big toe, and cold extremities.

5. THE HEART CHANNEL OF THE HAND (SHAOYIN)

The Heart Channel of the Hand (Shaoyin) begins in the heart, descends internally past the diaphragm, and connects with the small intestine. A branch from the heart region, runs upward along the side of the throat, and passes through the pharynx; connecting with the tongue and the eye. Then traveling laterally to connect with the ear.

The original channel ascends from the heart region to the lung, and emerges superficially in the middle of the axilla (armpit). Then traveling along the back of the middle of the upper arm, passing behind the Lung Channel of the Hand (Taiyin), and the Pericardium Channel of the Hand (Jueyin). Going downward to the rear border of the middle of the forearm, and to the center of the wrist. Then to the palm, and traveling along the middle of the palm to the smallest finger. Finally, connecting with the Shaoze point on the small finger to connect with Small Intestine Meridian of the Hand (Taiyang).

Careful and correct stimulation of this channel may help relieve: Psychosis, epilepsy, insomnia, and cardiovascular diseases such as tachycardia (sped up heart rate), bradycardia (slowed heart rate), angina pectoris (Cramping pain in the chest). Other conditions treatable would be: Dry throat, pain in the chest (above the heart), excessive thirst, cold hands and feet, and painful or hot and sweaty palms.

FIGURE A-5

The Heart Channel of Hand-*Shaoyin*

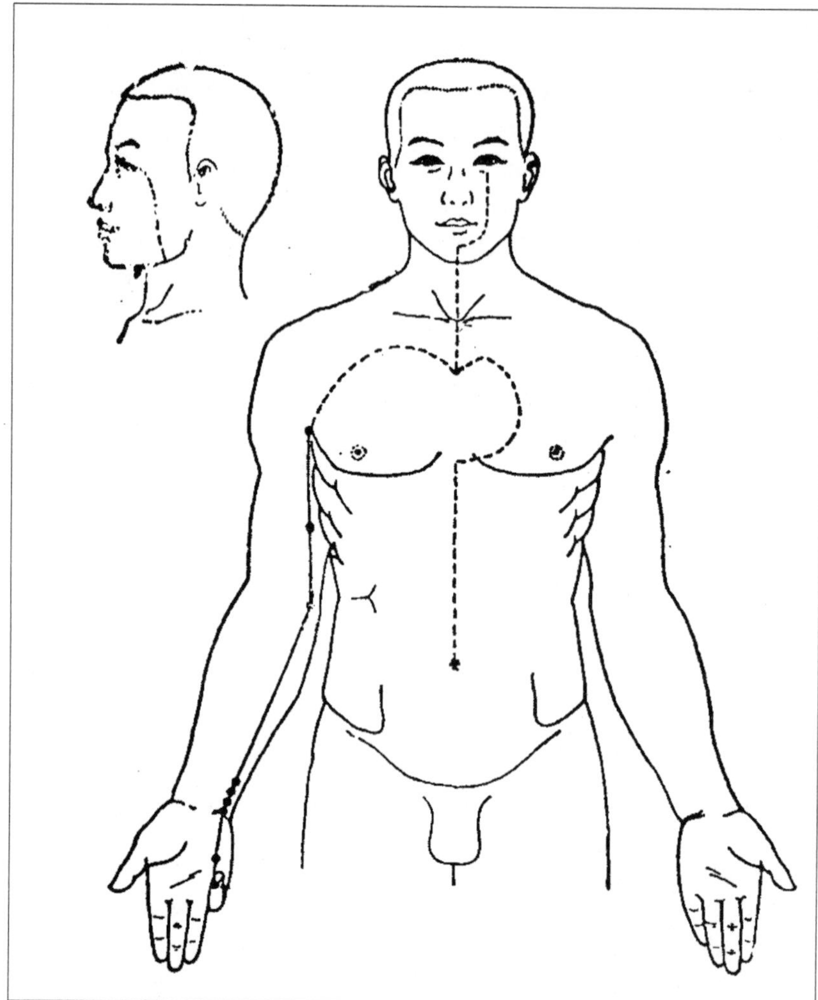

6. THE SMALL INTESTINE CHANNEL OF THE HAND (TAIYANG)

This channel starts from the tip of the small finger at the Shaoze point and passes through the hand, ascends to the wrist, and then proceeds through the forearm. Then traveling along the middle of the arm bone, and to the side of the upper arm. Going out of the shoulder joint, circling round the shoulder blade, and continues forward to above the clavicle where the channel divides into two branches.

An Internal branch descends from above the clavicle into the chest and connects with the heart. Then runs parallel with the esophagus, descends past the diaphragm, and continues past the stomach. Passing through the small intestine, and joining the Xiajuxu point on the Stomach Channel of the Foot (Yangming).

A superficial branch ascends from above the clavicle along the side of the neck. Continues along the cheek, reaches the side of the nose, and ends at the inner corner of the eye. Finally, the chan-

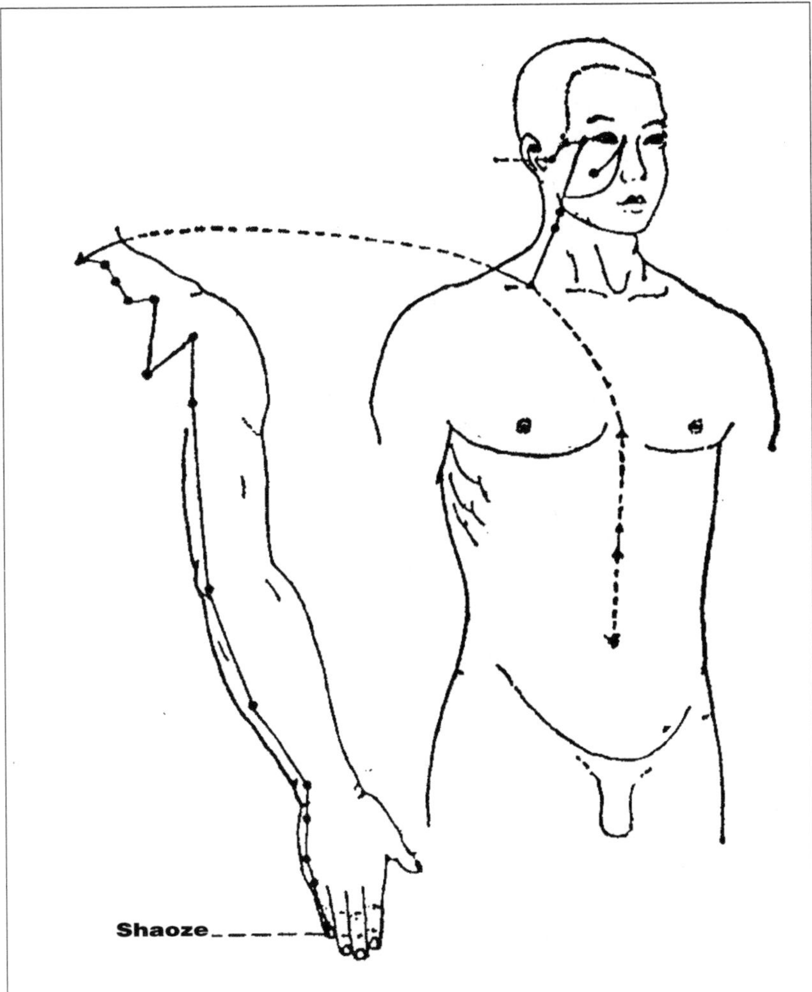

FIGURE A-6
The Small Intestine Channel of Hand-*Taiyang*

nel distributes obliquely over the cheek bone, and connects with the Jingming point on the Urinary Bladder Channel of the Foot (Taiyang).

Careful and correct stimulation of this channel may help relieve: Sore throat, stiff neck, impaired hearing, back pain, scapula pain, pains on the side of the neck, shoulders, upper arms, elbows, and forearms.

7. THE URINARY BLADDER OF THE FOOT (TAIYANG)

The Urinary Bladder of the Foot (Taiyang) commences at the Jingming point at the inner corner of the eye, ascends to the forehead, and continues up to the top of the head. There a branch splits off and goes to above the ear. The original channel leaves the top of the head for the brain and then comes out and runs down to the back of the neck. There at the nape of the neck the channel splits into two branches:

FIGURE A-7
The Urinary Bladder Channel of Foot-*Taiyang*

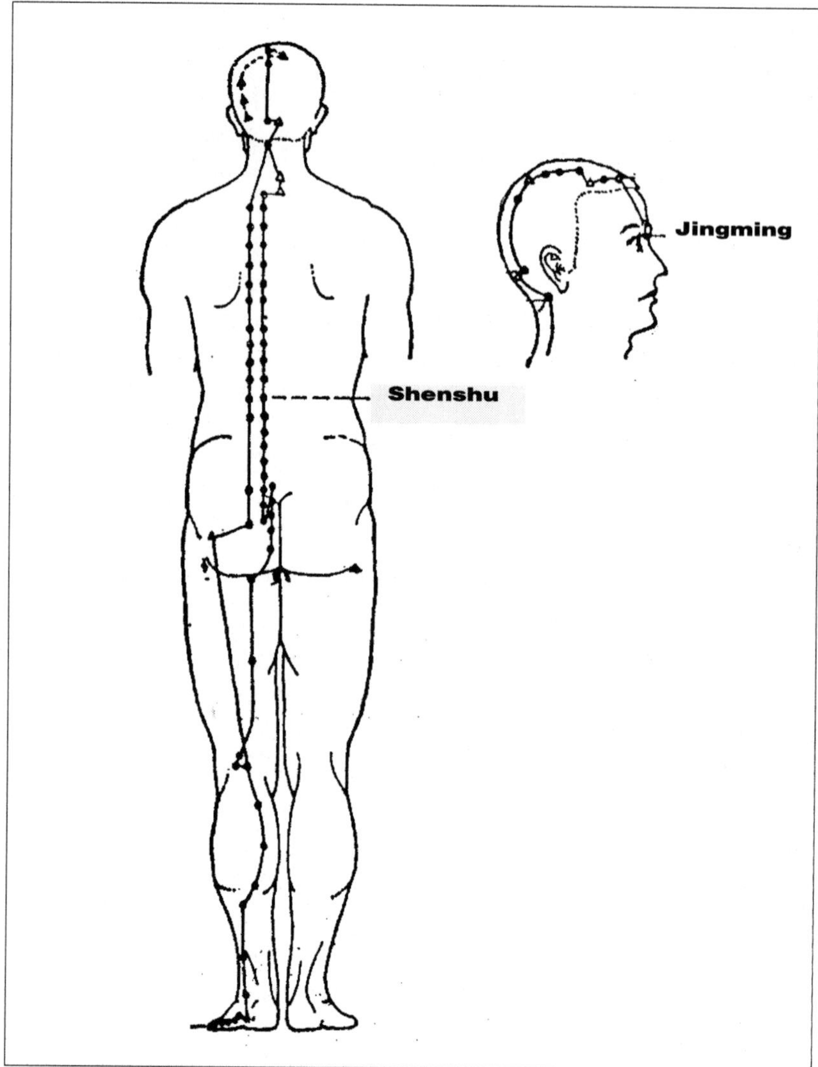

A middle branch continues along the middle of the scapula (Shoulder blade), travels parallel with the spinal column down to the lumbar region to the Shenshu point. Then continues to the loins, enters the abdomen from the kidney area, connects with the kidney, and passes through the urinary bladder. Exiting the kidney area, descending the buttocks, turning upward to the first rear opening between the vertebrae in the pelvic region where the nerves pass, and descends to the fourth opening between the vertebrae in the pelvic region where the nerves pass. Then travels downward and sideways to meet the lateral branch.

A lateral branch descends from the nape of the neck, down the back parallel with and outside the middle branch, and continues down to the Huantiao point where it intersects with the Gallbladder Channel of the Foot (Shaoyang). Continuing along the thigh, meeting the middle branch near the knee level. Descending along the back of the calf, through the back of the side of the ankle, and continues along the side of the foot to the small toe. Finally, traveling obliquely to the center of the ball of the foot, and to the Yongquan point of the Kidney Channel of the Foot (Shaoyin).

Careful and correct stimulation of this channel may help relieve: Headaches that have the feeling of the Chi rushing upwards, pain and diseases in the eyes, head, nape of the neck, back, lumbar, and sacral regions. Hemorrhoids, malaria, insanity, epilepsy, epistaxis, pains in the foot, and dysfunction of the small toes are associated with tendon trouble caused by dysfunction of the Urinary Channel of the Foot (Taiyang).

FIGURE A-8

The Kidnay Channel of Foot-*Saoyin*

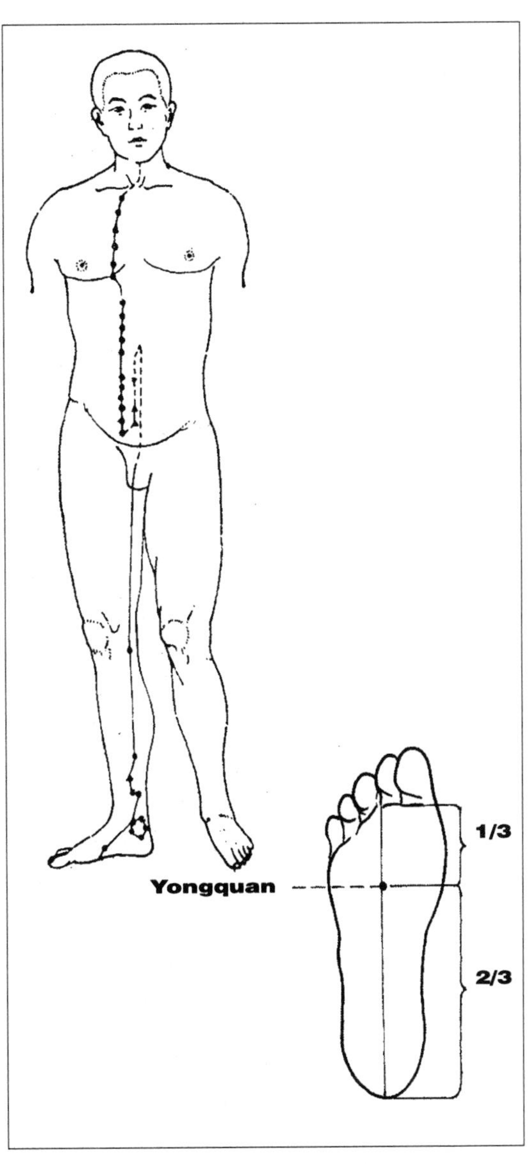

8. THE KIDNEY CHANNEL OF THE FOOT (SHAOYIN)

This channel begins on the bottom of the tip of the small toe and travels obliquely towards the center of the ball of the foot to the Yongquan point. Emerging and continuing to the ankle, and reaching the heel. Ascending from the heel, intersecting the Spleen Channel of the Foot (Taiyin), continuing to ascend along the middle of the leg and thigh to meet the Huiyin point of the Ren Meridian, and passes the anus. Continuing up to the lumbar, to the Mingmen (Life Gate) point on the Du Meridian, and going internally to pass through the kidney. Then descends from the kidney to connect with the urinary bladder.

It's direct branch comes back out of the kidney, runs straight up from the liver and diaphragm into the lung. Then traveling to the throat and terminating in the root of the tongue.

Another branch exits the lung connecting with the heart, spreading through the chest, and connects with the Pericardium channel of the Hand (Jueyin).

Careful and correct stimulation of this channel may help relieve: chest pains, insomnia, mental disease, hunger without a taste for food, bronchial wheezing, blurred

FIGURE A-9
The Pericardium Channel of Hand-*Jueyin*

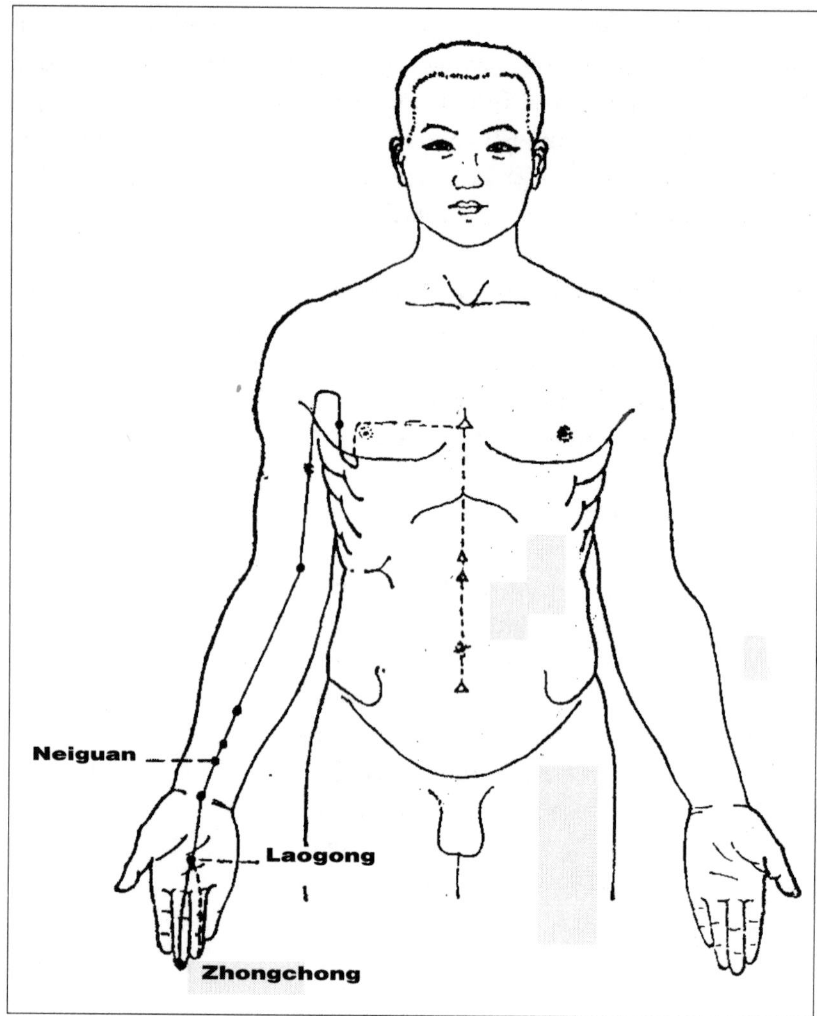

vision, nervousness, burning sensation of the mouth, dry tongue, swollen throat, jaundice, dysentery, pains in the spine, thighs, and burning sensations on the soles of the feet.

9. THE PERICARDIUM CHANNEL OF THE HAND (JUEYIN)

This channel begins in the chest where it exits and then enters the Pericardium. Then it descends through the diaphragm, and connects with the triple warmers in the upper, middle, and lower areas of the body. Traverses from the Pericardium, and follows the middle of the upper arm, turning downward between the Lung and Heart Channels. Then travels along the midline of the biceps muscle, enters the elbow, continuing down the forearm, passing through the Neiguan point, and the wrist. Finally, going into the palm to the Laogong point, and continues to the tip of the middle finger to the Zhongchong point.

A small branch from the Laogong point runs along the tip of the ring finger to the Guanchong point, and there links with the Triple Warmer Channel of the Hand (Shaoyang).

Careful and correct stimulation of this channel may help relieve: Hot and sweaty palms, cardiovascular disease, chest pain, insomnia, and mental disease.

10. THE TRIPLE WARMER CHANNEL OF THE HAND (SHAOYANG)

This channel originates at the Guanchong point at the tip of the ring finger. Running upward through the fourth and fifth metacarpal bones, and along the back of the wrist. Traveling along

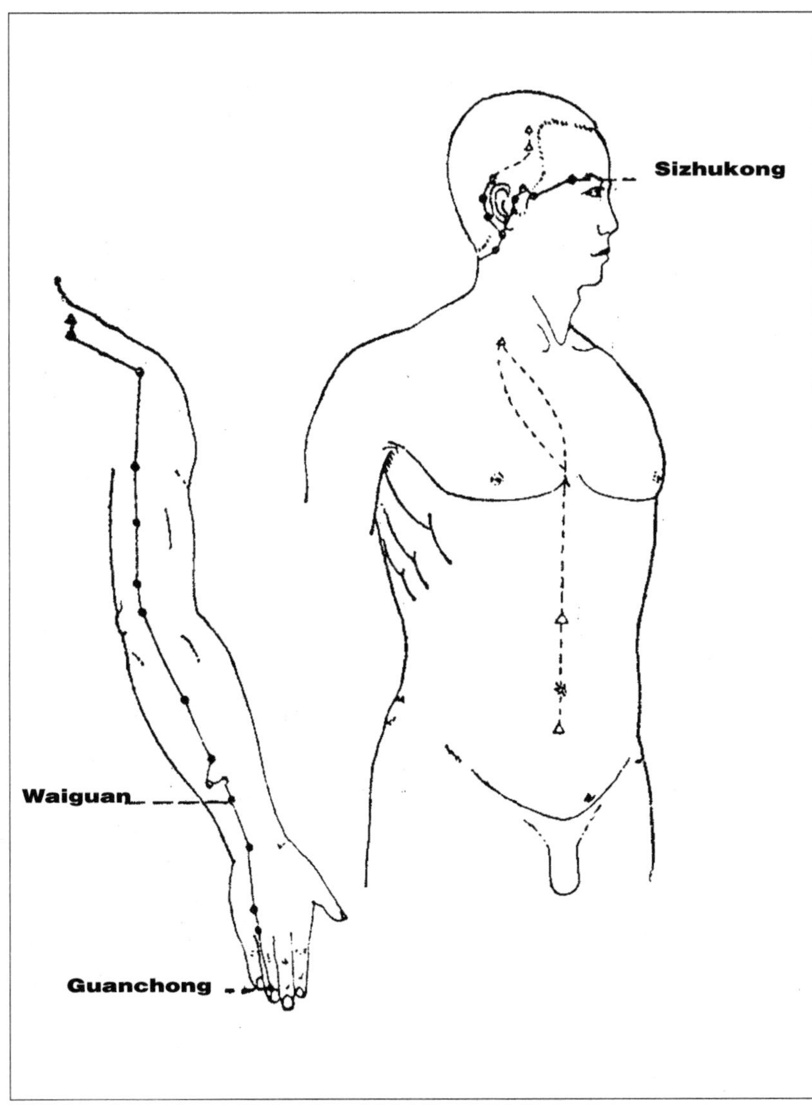

FIGURE A-10
The Triple-warmer Channel of Hand-*Shaoyang*

the forearm between the radius and the ulna through the Waiguan point. Ascends through the point of the elbow, and continues along the upper arm to the shoulder area. There it meets the Gallbladder Channel and the Du Meridian. Then winds over to above the clavicle, and spreads through the chest. Connecting with the Shanzhong (or, Tanzhong) point of the Ren Meridian (located between the two nipples). Also there mingling with the Pericardium. Descending through the diaphragm it reaches the Triple Warmer, and connects

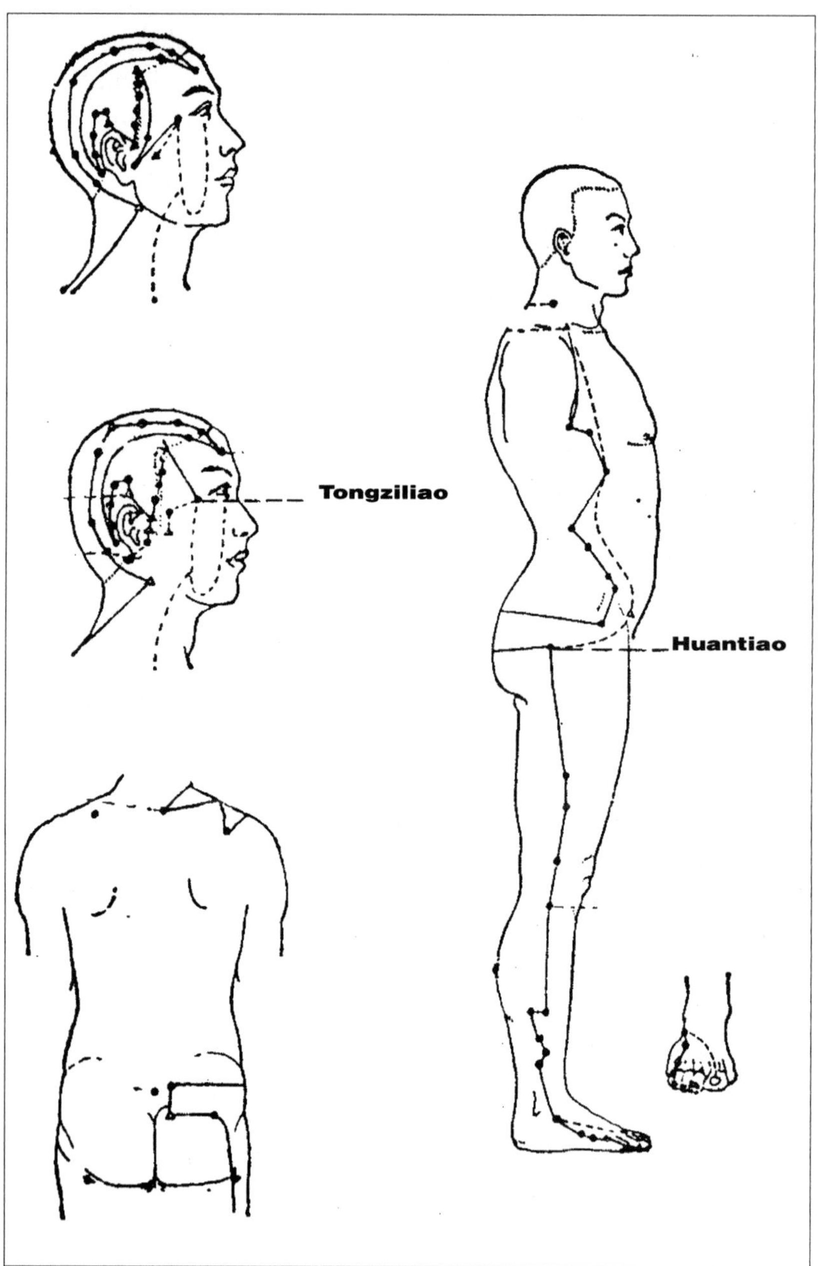

FIGURE A-11
The Gall Bladder Channel of Foot-*Shaoyan*

in succession with the upper, middle, and lower portions of the body. One of it's branches ascends from the Shanzhong point to above the clavicle, goes upward to the nape of the neck. Then traveling to the ear, and curves down the cheek.

Another branch originates outside the ear, and goes into the ear. Exits in front of the ear and crosses the upper cheek, and through the Sizhukong point to the outer corner of the eye at the Tongziliao point on the Gallbladder Channel of the Foot (Shaoyang).

Careful and correct stimulation of this channel may help relieve: Deafness, swelling of the pharynx, sore throat, cheek pains, and pain in the outer corner of the eye.

11. THE GALL BLADDER CHANNEL OF THE FOOT (SHAOYANG)

This channel begins at the outer corner of the eye at the Tongziliao point. Turns upward at the corner of the forehead, then descends to the ear, and continues running along side of the neck in front of the Triple Warmer Channel to the shoulder. Then turning backwards it moves behind the Triple Warmer Channel, and enters the body above the clavicle.

One branch originates outside the ear, passes through the ear, comes out in front of the ear, and reaches the outer corner of the eye.

Another branch leaves the outer corner of the eye, descends and continues down through the cheek, and meets the original branch above the clavicle. Then descends through the chest, diaphragm, liver, and enters the gall bladder. Then travels inside the hypochondriac region, runs superficially across the pubic hair, and goes transversely into the hip to the Huantiao point.

A third branch descends from above the collar bone to the axilla (armpit), runs down the lateral aspect of the chest, and continues down to the hip to meet the previous branch at the Huantiao point. There it continues to descend along the side of the thigh, to the knee, along the front of the fibula (calf bone). Descending further, and coming out in front of the ankle bone, continuing along the bottom of the foot, through the first and second metacarpal bones. Finally to the bone at the tip of the big toe to the Dadun point where it connects with the Liver Channel of the Foot (Jueyin).

Careful and correct stimulation of this channel may help relieve: Migraines, deafness, liver and gallbladder diseases, bitter taste in the mouth, constant sighing, sallow complexion, hot feet, and pains along the course of the channel.

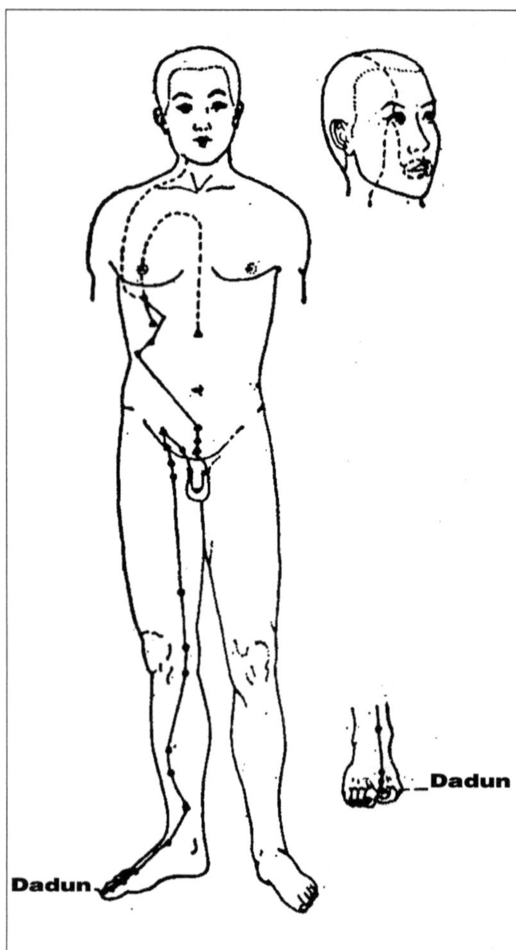

FIGURE A-12
The Liver Channel of the Foot-*Jueyin*

12. THE LIVER CHANNEL OF THE FOOT (JUEYIN)

The Liver Channel of the Foot (Jueyin starts in the big toe at the Dadun point, runs upward along the middle of the foot to near the ankle bone where it crosses the Spleen Channel of the Foot (Taiyin), then runs behind the Spleen Channel. Running further upward to the middle of the knee, along the middle of the thigh, through the pubic hair region to join the Spleen Channel. Curves around the genitalia, ascends the lower abdomen, joining the Ren Meridian, and then ascends obliquely to the stomach. Curving around the stomach, the channel then enters the liver, connects with the gall-bladder, and continues to ascend to the diaphragm. Passing through the diaphragm, it spreads over the ribs, and then ascends along the back of the throat to the nasal passage where it connects with the surrounding tissues of the eye. Coming out of the forehead, and connects with the Du Meridian. Then going into the brain, and up to the ear.

One branch originates in the tissues connecting the eyeball with the brain, goes down into the cheek, and curves around the inside of the lips.

Another branch arises from the liver, passes through the diaphragm, and spreads upward to the lung, where it connects with the Lung Channel of the Hand (Taiyang) and completes the circulation of the twelve channels.

Careful and correct stimulation of this channel may help relieve: Headache, inability to bend, swollen and painful testes, psychosis, eye diseases, epilepsy, vomiting, watery diarrhea, mal absorption, and bed wetting.

SYSTEMIC CIRCULATION

When the Chi flows in all twelve channels without any hindrance or stoppage, this is known as the "Systemic Circulation." Achieving the Systemic Circulation is not as difficult as it may seem. Continued employment of the natural forces of motion with natural breathing (or, gentle breathing that is taken as needed and harmonized with movements), instead of isolated force or the holding of breath, will encourage all the channels to be open and the flow of chi stimulated.

B. EIGHT MERIDIANS

Aside from the twelve channels there are eight meridians. While the twelve channels are seen as routes, the eight meridians are often seen as reservoirs. They have their own special routes, and do not necessarily follow a set pattern as described so sequentially as the twelve channels.

When the Chi is flowing in all of the 12 channels, this is called the "Systemic Circulation." When the Chi is overflowing on the channels, then the eight meridians are utilized to store this excess of flow and recirculate the Chi on the twelve channels as required. However, when there isn't a sufficient amount of Chi on the twelve channels, then the eight meridians are called upon to deliver the Chi necessary or support the body's vital functions. Therefore the eight channels help maintain the circulation along the twelve channels.

The eight meridians are as follows: Du (Back Midline), Ren (Front Midline), Chong (Center of Body, Flushing), Dai (Belt), Yinqiao (The Yin Heel), Yangqiao (The Yang Heel), Yinwei (The Yin Link), and Yangwei (The Yang Link). See Figures B1-B8 for illustrations and descriptions of the 8 meridians.

1. THE DU MERIDIAN (OR, DUMAI; BACK MIDLINE)

Also known as the Governor Vessel, the Du Meridian goes along the back midline. It has broad connections through it's branches (connecting with three Yang Channels of the Foot and Hand; as well as the Yangwei Meridian), and because it is located mostly on the back of the body (which is considered Yang), it is known as the "Sea of All Yang Vessels."

The Du meridian originates in the lower abdomen and comes out the perineum to curve around the anus, and ascends through the Changqiang point which is the first point on the meridian. Continuing up the midline of the back through the Mingmen (Life Gate) point, and continues upward towards the neck. Passing through the Dazhui point located at the neck bone between C7 and T1. Continuing up the nape of the neck, where it goes into the brain. Then passes over the top of the head at the Baihui point. Continues over the head, to the forehead, and over the column of the nose. Finally, terminating at the Yinjiao point.

Careful and correct stimulation of this meridian may help

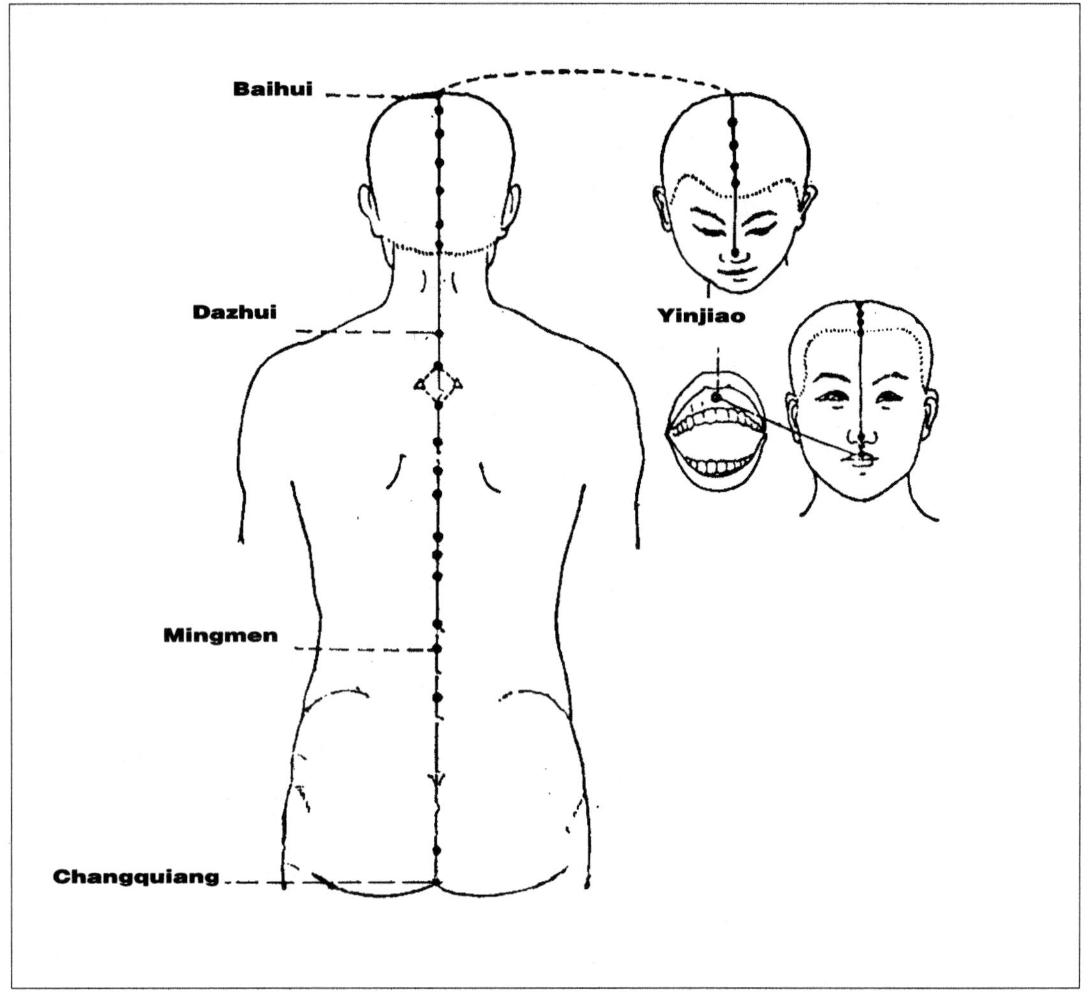

FIGURE B-1
The *Du* Meridian

relieve: Rigid spine, shock, fever, coma, impotence, premature ejaculation, psychosis, and digestive diseases.

2. THE REN MERIDIAN (OR, REN MAI; FRONT MIDLINE)

Also known as the Conception Vessel, the Ren Meridian begins in the lower abdomen and emerges at the Huiyin point (between the scrotum/vagina and anus) then flows over the external genitalia and connects with the genital organ. Goes upward through the pubic hair region. Ascending through the abdomen passing through the Qihai point, the Shenque point (or, Navel), and through the Shanzhong point (Center of Breast Bone). Continues up to the throat, to the lower jaw bone where it turns around the lips and finalizes at the Chengjiang point located below the bottom lip.

Careful and correct stimulation of this meridian may help relieve: Sterility, hernia, acute sore throat, urogenital (urinary and genital) diseases, profuse vomiting or diarrhea.

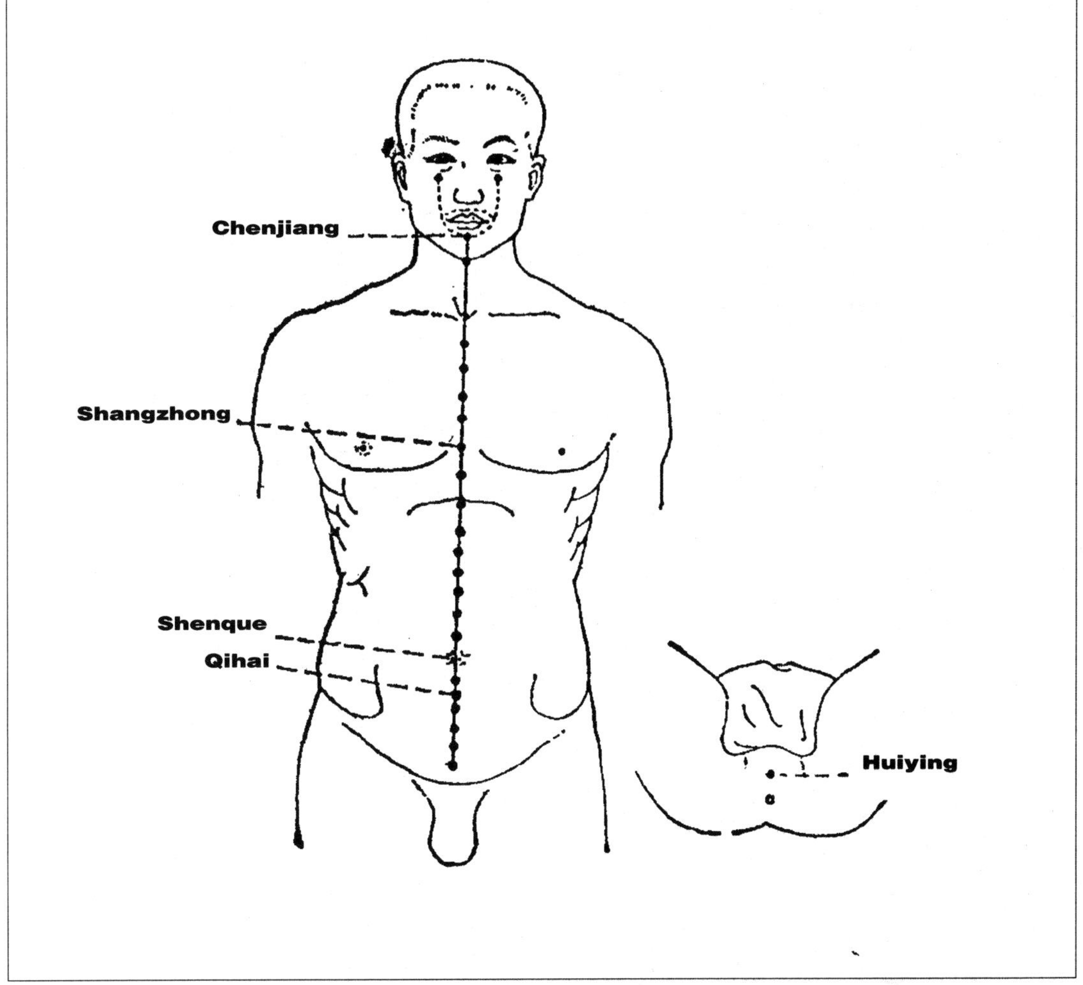

FIGURE B-2
The *Ren* Meridian

PULMONARY CIRCULATION (CONNECTING DU AND REN MERIDIANS)

In addition to the Systemic Circulation, which is the Chi flowing and circulating along all 12 channels, the other important circulation is the Pulmonary Circulation. A smaller circulation than the Systemic, the Pulmonary Circulation is an orbit of energy achieved by connecting and circulating the chi without stopping along the Du and Ren meridians.

The Du meridian (Figure B-1) begins at the Changqiang point, and flows up the exterior mid back line, over the head, down over the nose to the Yinjiao point (Located on the frenulum of the upper lip, which is that part that connects the upper lip to the gum.). The Ren meridian (Figure B-2) begins at the Huiying point which is located between the scrotum/vagina and the anus. Running up the mid front line of the body to the Chengjiang point located in the center below the bottom lip and above the chin.

FIGURE B-3
The *Chong* Meridian

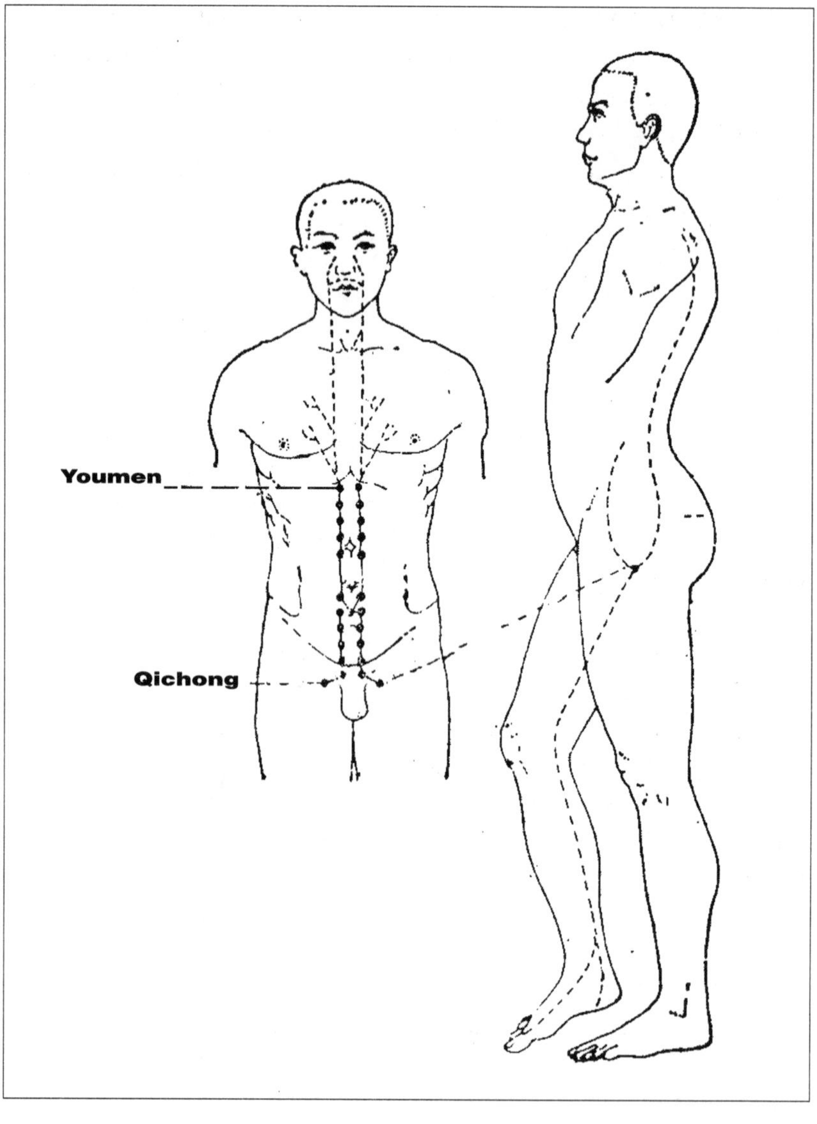

Youmen
Qichong

In order for these two channels to be connected (since the mouth creates a space between the Yinjiao and Chengjiang), bring the teeth together, and let the tongue gently touch the upper palate. Thereby connecting these two vital meridians, and making way for the Pulmonary Circulation.

However, the practitioner is cautioned not to concentrate too much on touching the tip of the tongue to the upper palate, in order to make the connection. Very often too much concentration on this can cause the Chi to stop at this point of connection and not circulate. Also if force is applied with the tongue to make the connection, then it is possible for the chi to become stuck at this point, and prevent the connection of the Du and Ren Meridians; as well as disallow the Pulmonary circulation.

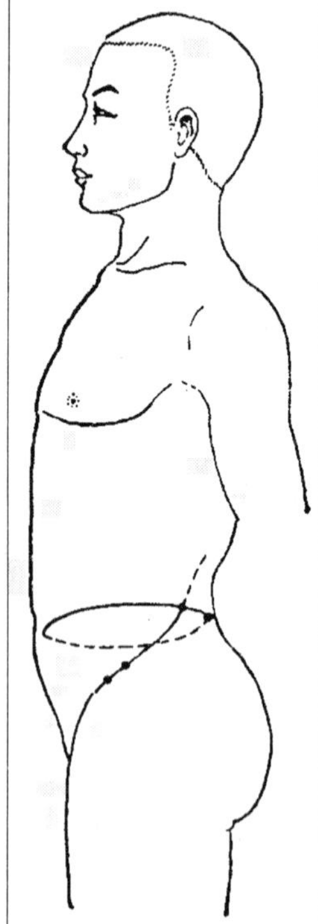

FIGURE B-4
The *Dai* Meridian

3. CHONG MERIDIAN (OR, CHONGMAI; CENTER OF BODY)

The Chong Meridian, also known as the Flush Vessel, controls and regulates the chi and blood inside the twelve regular channels. It originates from the inside of the lower abdomen and emerges at the Huiying point. Ascends through the center of the spinal column.

The superficial branch of the meridian passes the Qichong point , meets with the Kidney channel of the Foot (Shaoyin), and ascends with it along both sides of the abdomen to the Youmen point where it spreads through the chest. Then runs through the throat up into the nasal cavity.

Careful and correct stimulation of this meridian may help relieve: Sterility, uterine bleeding, abnormal rising of chi, spasm in abdomen, spitting blood, stuffiness in the chest, chest pain, and chest pain or upper abdomen spasm with diarrhea.

4. THE DAI MERIDIAN (OR, DAIMAI; BELT LINE)

The Dai Meridian, also known as the Belt Vessel (because it runs transversely around the waist like a belt), binds together all the channels of the body. The Dai Meridian is activated most often when turning the waist during practice. The Dai Meridian originates just below the ribs, and descends obliquely to the Daimai point the 26th Point on the Gall Bladder Channel, and runs transversely around the waist (at the level of the second lumbar vertebra).

Careful and correct stimulation of this meridian may help relieve: Abdominal tension, soreness and inability to turn the waist , numbness of the limbs, and menstrual disorders.

5. THE YANGQIAO MERIDIAN (OR, YANGQIAOMAI; YANG HEEL LINE)

The Yangqiao Meridian, also known as the Yang Heel Vessel, controls the Yang Chi on the left and right sides of the entire body. The Yangqiao Meridian originates at the Shenmai point located on the side of the heel and runs to the Pushen point. From the Pushen point, it ascends along the ankle bone, passes the back border of the fibula (calf bone), and continues along the side of the thigh. Continues to ascend along the back side of the chest (above the heart), through the armpit fold, and then winds over through the

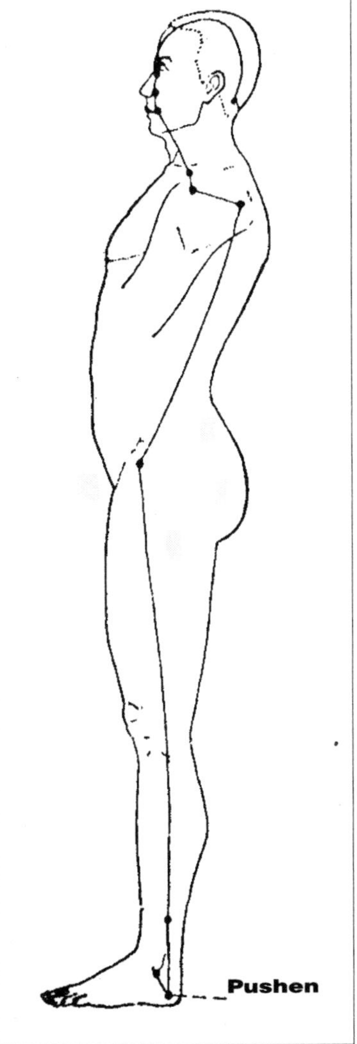

FIGURE B-5
The *Yangqiao* Meridian

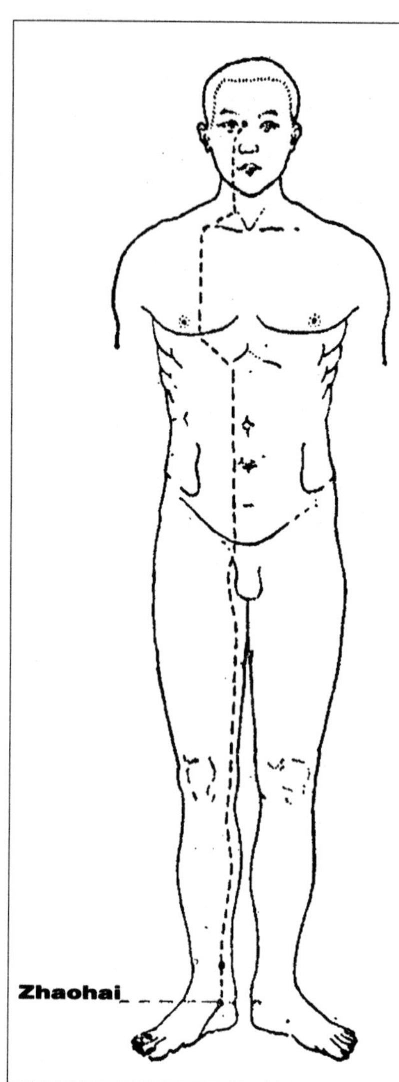

FIGURE B-6

The *Yingiao* Meridian

shoulder. Then ascends along the neck to the corner of the mouth, continues up to the inner corner of the eye, and up passed the forehead to the hairline. Continues over the side of the head to behind the ear and to the Fengchi point.

Careful and correct stimulation of this meridian may help relieve: Numbness of the hands and feet, headache, redness and pains in the eye, rigid and painful back, insomnia, and pain in the inner corner of the eye.

6. THE YINQIAO MERIDIAN (OR, YINQIAOMAI; YIN HEEL LINE)

The Yinqiao Meridian, also known as the Yin Heel Vessel, controls not only the Yin Chi on the left and right sides of the whole body, but is also associated with the opening and closing of the eyelids as well as the motion of the lower limbs. The Yinqiao Meridian runs almost parallel with Yangqiao Meridian on the inside of the legs.

The Yinqiao Meridian begins at the Zhaohai point on the foot. Ascends to the upper portion of the middle of the ankle bone, ascends the middle of the back of the legs, and straight to the external genitalia. Then continues to ascend along the abdomen and the chest to above the clavicle. Runs then along the throat , and the middle of the cheek bone. Finally reaches the inner corner of the eye where it meets the Yangqiao Meridian; as well as the Taiyang channels of the Hand and Foot.

Careful and correct stimulation of this meridian may help relieve: Dribbling urine, throat trouble, abdominal tension, and fullness and stuffiness in the chest.

7. THE YANGWEI MERIDIAN (OR, YANGWEIMAI; THE YANG LINK)

The Yangwei Meridian, also known as the Yang Linking Vessel, serves to maintain and communicate by distributing, regulating, and storing the chi and blood with all the Yang channels of the body. The Yangwei Meridian originates in the heel, and emerges from the ankle bone and runs upward, ascends along the Gallbladder Channel of the Foot Shaoyang, and passes through the hip. Further ascends upward along the back of the chest (above the

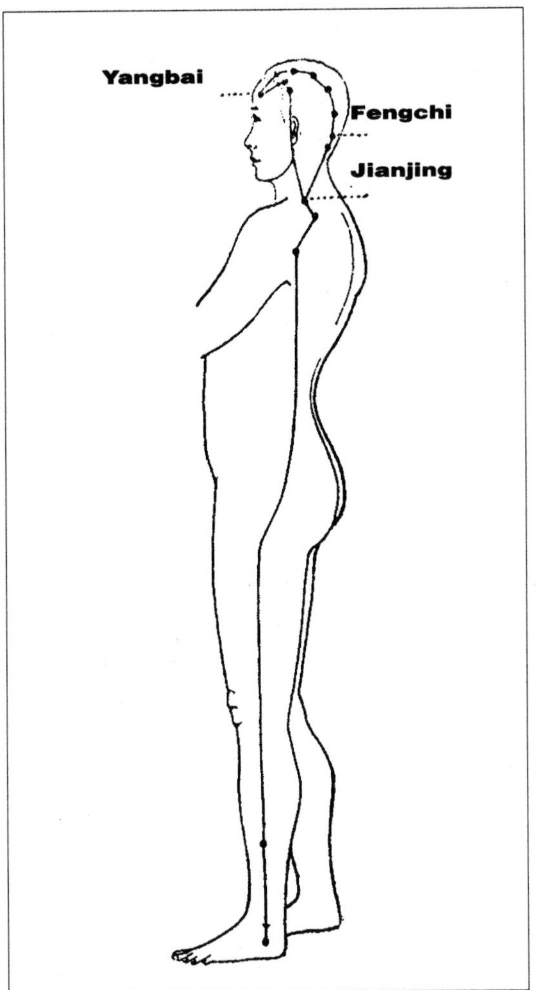

FIGURE B-7

The *Yangwei* Meridian

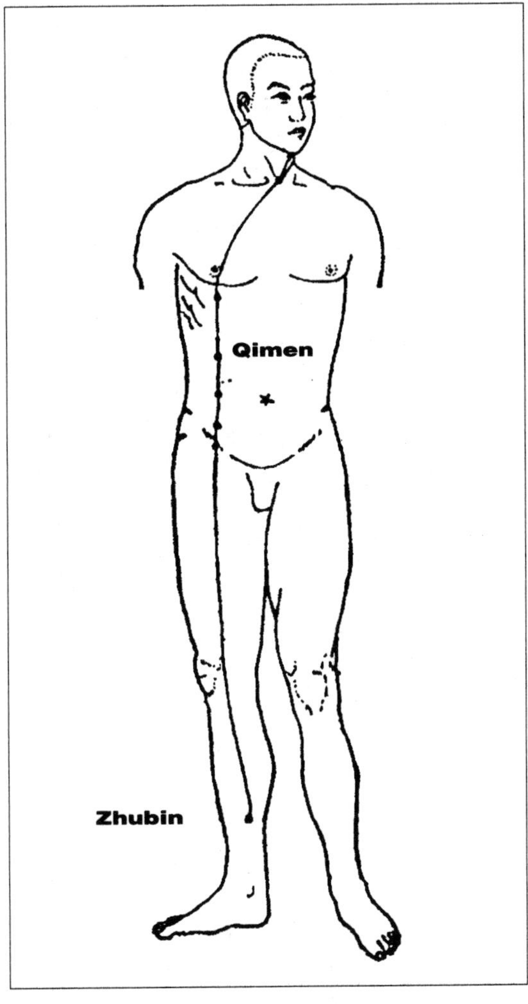

FIGURE B-8

The *Yinwei* Meridian

heart), travels along the back of the armpit to the shoulder, and through the base of the neck at the Jianjing point. Then traveling up past the ear, over to the Yangbai point on the forehead, and ascending up slightly on the side of the head. Continuing over the head and then descending through the Fengchi point, and ending at the Yamen point.

Careful and correct stimulation of this meridian may help relieve: Alternating spells of chill and fever, paralysis of the lower limbs, coldness of the knees, rigidness and pain in the back of the neck, headache, and colds.

8. THE YINWEI MERIDIAN (OR, YINWEIMAI; THE YIN LINK)

The Yinwei Meridian, also known as the Yin Linking Vessel,

serves to maintain and communicate by distributing, regulating, and storing the chi and blood with all the Yin channels of the body. The Yinwei Meridian originates at the Zhubin point on the middle of the leg. Ascends along the middle of the leg through the thigh, and the middle of the lower extremities passing through the Qimen point. Nearing the nipple it continues to ascend and transverses the chest, and then passes through the throat and the root of the tongue.

Careful and correct stimulation of this meridian may help relieve: Cardiac pain, stomach ache, pain in the chest and the portion of the chest above the heart, and diarrhea.

C. THE THREE DANTIANS

In our study of the Wild Goose Chi Kung we will concern our-

FIGURE C

The Three Dantians

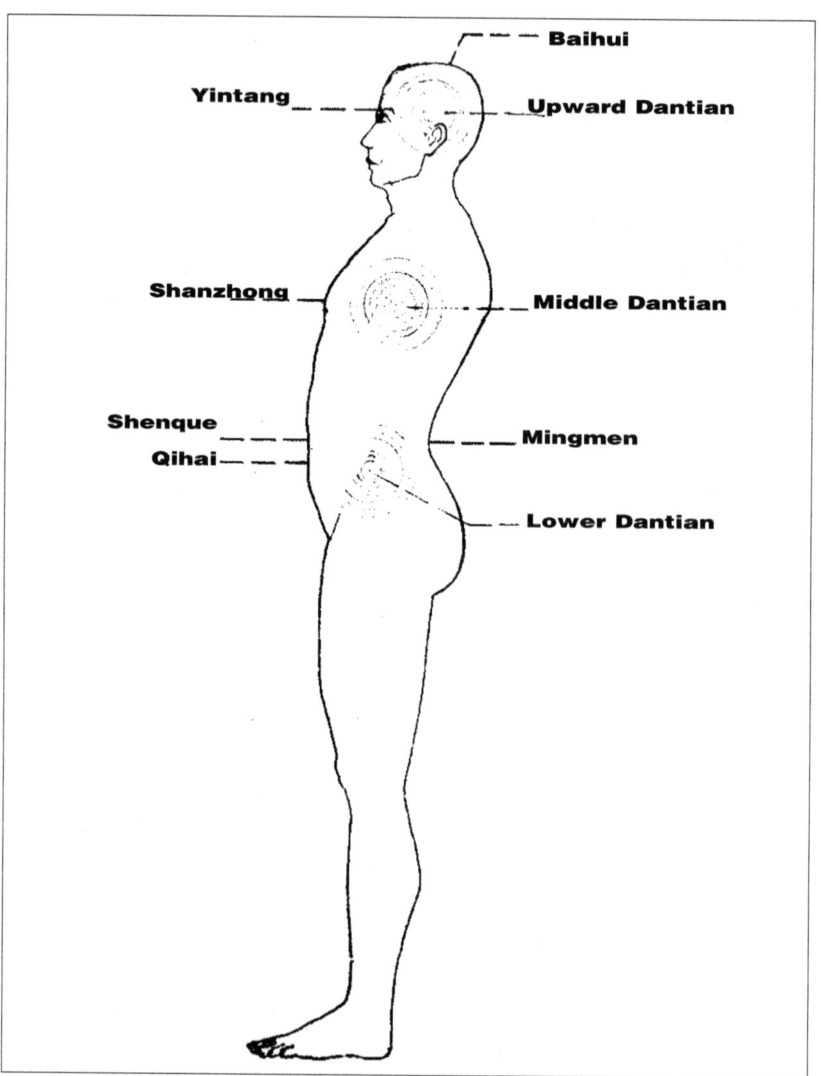

selves with three sensitive areas known as Dantians. Gently massaging or utilizing the hands at close distance to the superficial aspects of the Dantians on the front of the body may help you to sensitize or locate your Three Dantians.

The Three Dantians are referred to as Upward, Middle, and Lower Dantian (See figure C-1). The Upward Dantian is located in the head area. The front and center of which is usually thought to be superficially located between the two eyebrows. The Middle Dantian is located between the shoulder blades and the breast area. The front and center of which is usually thought to be superficially located between the nipples in the center of the breast bone. The Lower Dantian is located in the lower abdomen and pelvic region, whose front and center point is thought to be superficially located about three fingers below the navel at the Qihai (Ironically known as the Chi Ocean) point.

Chi is collected at these three areas, and ultimately brought down and stored in the Lower Dantian. The Lower Dantian can be thought of as a "Chi Bank" where deposits and withdrawals of energy are made.

When you finish your Chi Kung practice, deposit the Chi you've developed from your practice, and deposit fresh Chi in the Lower Dantian. Saving Chi to ward off stress and disease as needed. When sick, your energy stored in your Lower Dantian is drawn upon to combat sickness. If you continue to draw on your "Chi Account" without depositing more Chi, you will have less and less. Continuing to withdraw without replacing more Chi will eventually create an overdraft or shortage of energy. If left unattended or cared for, serious sickness or disease may develop.

This is why regardless of the type of Chi Kung you practice, when you are done practicing you need to store what Chi you have developed in your Lower Dantian. Making a deposit of fresh Chi you have worked for in your practice.

D. ACU-MERIDIAN POINTS IN WILD GOOSE CHI KUNG

For our study of the Wild Goose Chi Kung we will concern ourselves with 21 points (See Figures D-1 through D-21). As with the three sensitive areas known as Dantians, gently, softly massaging or utilizing your hands at a close distance to sensitize yourself to the points is suggested, in order to begin to discover the general area or precise location of your points as utilized in Chi Kung practice.

Again the locations of the points will have some variance from individual to individual. As our physical features and bone struc-

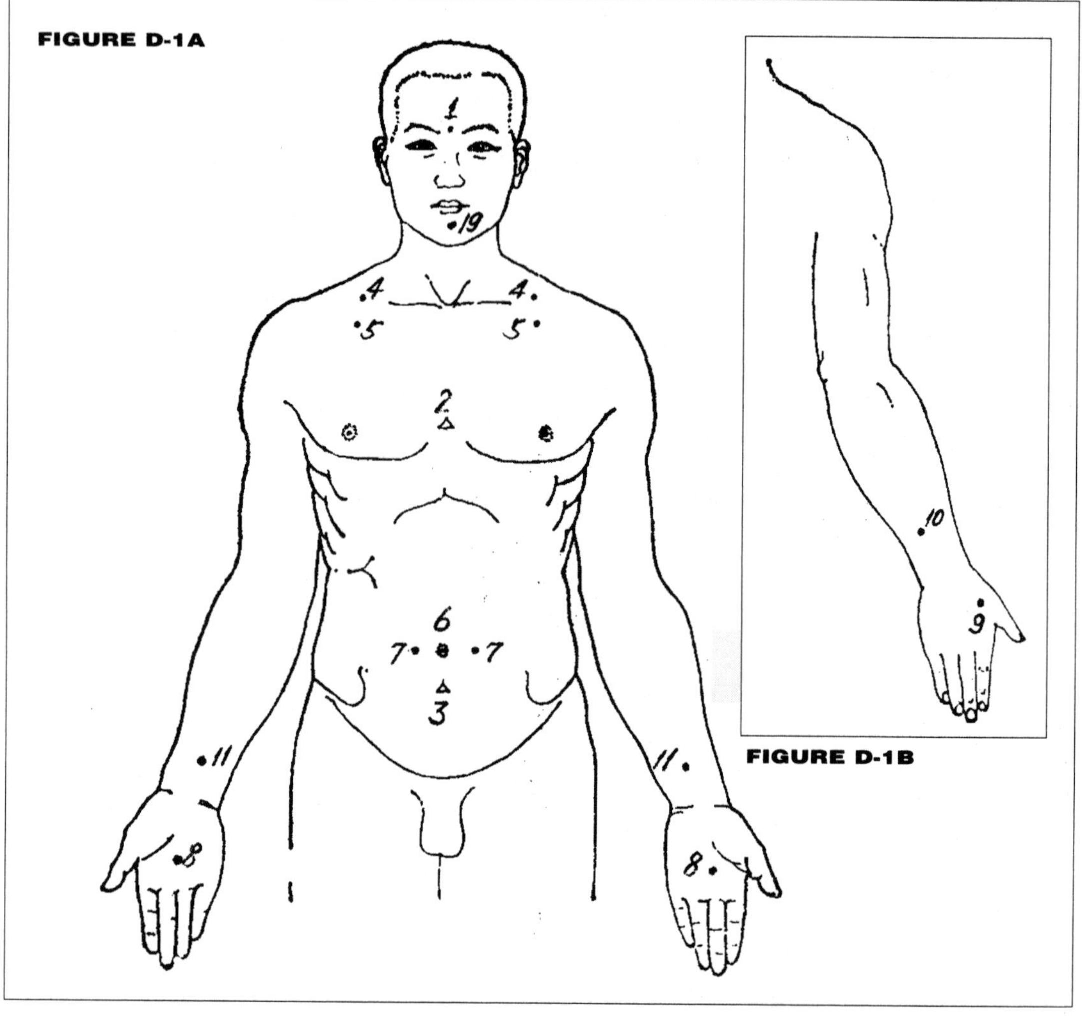

tures vary, so does the precise location of our points.

The points with basic information about each one that we will refer to in Wild Goose Chi Kung are: Yintang, Shanzhong (also known as Tanzhong), Qihai, Quepen, Qihu, Shenque (also known as Shenjue), Tianshu, Laogong, Hegu, Waiguan, Neiguan, Dazhui, Mingmen, Shenshu, Huantiao,Baihui, Taiyang, Yinjiao, Chengjiang,Yongquan, and Huiying.

1. YINTANG

The Yintang point is located between the eyebrows in the center of the frontal and superficial parameters of the Upward Dantian. The Yintang point is an unusual point in that it is not located on any channel or meridian. These types of unusual points are often referred to as extra points. The Yintang is often referred to as extra point number 1. Careful and correct stimulation of this point can stimulate fresh blood flow to the head area, correct low blood pressure, or correct deficiency of vital energy.

2. SHANZHONG
("MIDDLE CHEST" ALSO CALLED TANZHONG)

Located on the Ren Meridian between the nipples in the center of the breast bone, the Shanzhong (also called Tanzhong) point is located in the center of the frontal and superficial parameters of the Middle Dantian. Careful and correct stimulation of this area point can correct deficiency of vital energy and can help correct an overactive menstrual cycle.

3. QIHAI ("CHI OCEAN")

Located on the Ren Meridian three fingers or so below the navel. The Qihai point is located at the center of the frontal and superficial parameters of the Lower Dantian. The Qihai, or "Chi Ocean," can be viewed as the gateway to the actual "Ocean of Chi" in the Lower Dantian. For any problem, concentration on this point is the safest. Careful and correct stimulation of this point can correct kidney energy problems. Remember, the Lower Dantian is where Chi is stored, created, fired, and delivered.

4. QUEPEN ("CENTER ABOVE COLLAR BONE")

Located on the Stomach channel, the Quepen point is located above the collar bone straight up from and on vertical alignment with the nipple on both sides of the body. Careful and correct stimulation (avoid deep pressure on this vital point) can relieve stress on the lymph glands, side effects of Tuberculosis, asthma, or hiccups.

5. QIHU ('CHI DOOR")

Located on the Stomach channel, the Qihu point is located below the Quepen point, below the collar bone, and straight up from and on vertical alignment with the nipple on both sides of the body. The Qihu, or "Chi Door," is an important point utilized in Wild Goose Chi Kung practice. Often Chi is poured in, or passes through the Qihu point on it's way down to the Lower Dantian for storage. Careful and correct stimulation can relieve asthmatic and bronchial conditions.

6. SHENQUE ("NAVEL," ALSO CALLED SHENJUE)

Located on the Ren meridian, the Shenque point is the navel. Careful and correct stimulation of this point can relieve intestinal infection, intestinal disorder, or diarrhea. Also helpful in relieving shock.

7. TIANSHU ("UPPER PIVOT")

Located on the Stomach channel, the Tianshu point is on the front of the body opposite the Shenshu point. Moreover, the Tianshu points can be found slightly outward on both sides of the Shenque (Navel) point. Careful and correct stimulation of this point can correct intestinal infection, constipation, and menstrual cramping.

8. LAOGONG ("PALACE OF LABOR")

Connected to the Pericardium channel, the Laogong point is found by curling the fingers into the center of the palm. Then where the middle finger contacts the space between the second and third metacarpal bones in the center of the palm, this is the Laogong point. Located in both palms, the Laogong point is also located straight through on the outside of both hands as well. Careful and correct stimulation at this point can help relieve cardiac pain and stroke complications, as well as stiffness of the tongue. The Laogong point is also a point where Chi can be emitted or received to and fro any direction, whether up, down, right, left, front or back.

9. HEGU ("CONNECTED VALLEYS")

Connected to the Large Intestine channel, the Hegu point is located in the fleshy area between the thumb and forefinger on the top of the hand on both hands. Careful and correct stimulation of this point can relieve headache, common cold, and palsy.

10. WAIGUAN ("OUTSIDE PASSAGE")

Located on the Triple Warmer channel, the Waiguan point is located opposite the Neiguan point on the outside of the arm near the wrist on both arms. Careful and correct stimulation of this point can relieve lung infection, common cold, and constipation.

11. NEIGUAN ("INSIDE PASSAGE")

Located on the Pericardium channel, the Neiguan point is located opposite the Waiguan point on the inside of the arm near the wrist on both arms. Careful and correct stimulation of this point is good for easing heart problems and stomach ache.

12. DAZHUI ("BIG VERTEBRA")

The Dazhui point is the Fourteenth point on the Du Meridian.

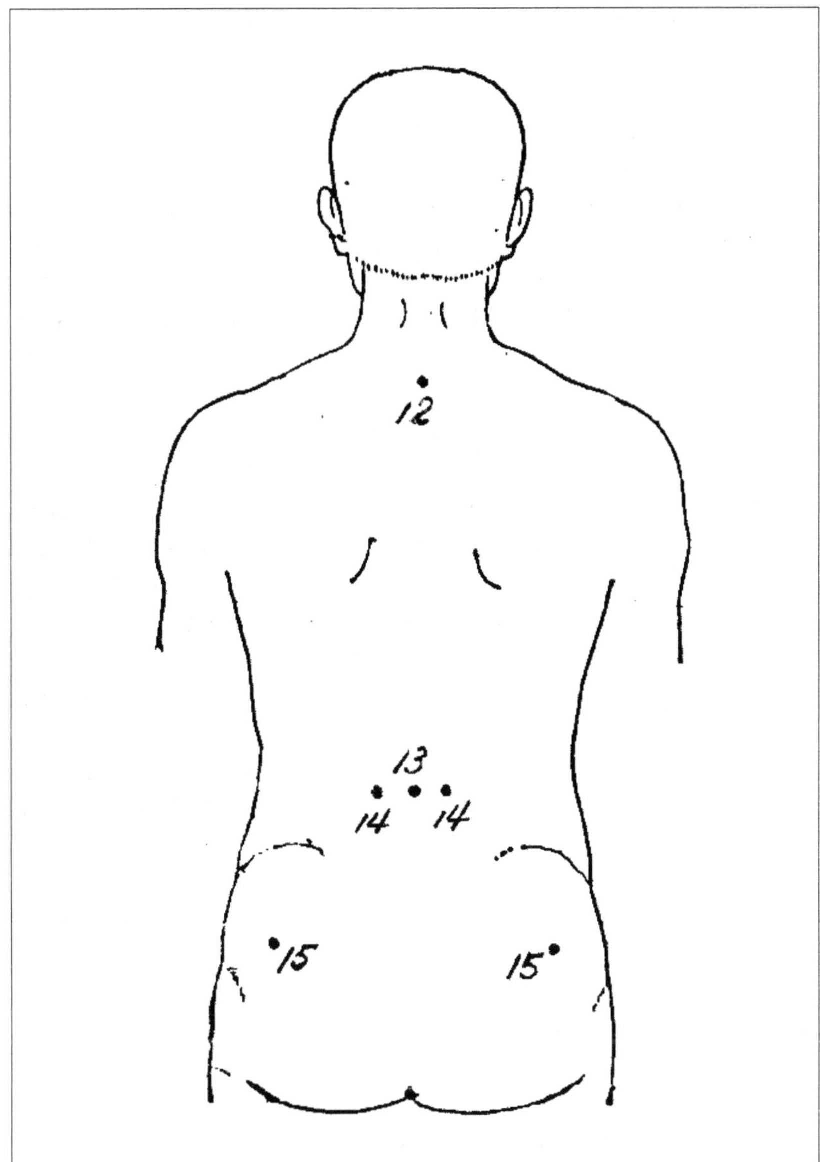

FIGURE D-2

Located on the neck bone, in the excavation below the seventh cervical vertebra. Careful and correct stimulation of this point can help relieve Asthma, colds, cough, fever, asthma, profuse sweating, and epilepsy.

13. MINGMEN ("LIFE GATE")

Located on the Du meridian, the Mingmen point is an important point found easily opposite your navel on your low back. Opening the Mingmen is essential in Chi Kung practice. Ancients tell that when a woman is far along in pregnancy, she needs to get under the baby with the strength of her legs, tucking her buttocks, and relaxing her hips in order to get about and continue to perform a day's work. If the woman could lower her center of gravity and get around, the birth of the child would not meet with any early complications. Instead, the ancients would say that the woman's Mingmen (Life Gate) is open, and that the child would likely be born healthy and strong. The body has a natural curve in the lower back. It's advantageous for the Chi Kung practitioner to lower their center of gravity, tuck the buttocks, flatten the back, and relax the hips. In order to open the vital Mingmen ("Life Gate") point to receive Fresh Chi and stimulate the channels and strengthen the vital organs.

Careful and correct stimulation can relieve impotence, involuntary seminal emission, and overcome menstrual disorders.

14. SHENSHU ("KIDNEY POINT")

Located on the Urinary Bladder channel, the Shenshu point is located on the back of the body opposite the Tianshu point. Moreover, the Shenshu points can be found slightly outward on both sides of the Mingmen in the low back. Careful and correct stimulation of this point can strengthen the kidneys, and help eliminate impotence, involuntary seminal emission, and help relieve or overcome menstrual disorders.

15. HUANTIAO ("CIRCULAR JUMP")

Located on the Gallbladder channel, the Huantiao point is located on the hip by the posterior (back) side of the femur on both hips. Careful and correct stimulation of this point can relieve Sciatica. Relieve pain in the lumbar region of the back, the thigh, and paralysis of the lower limb.

FIGURE D-3

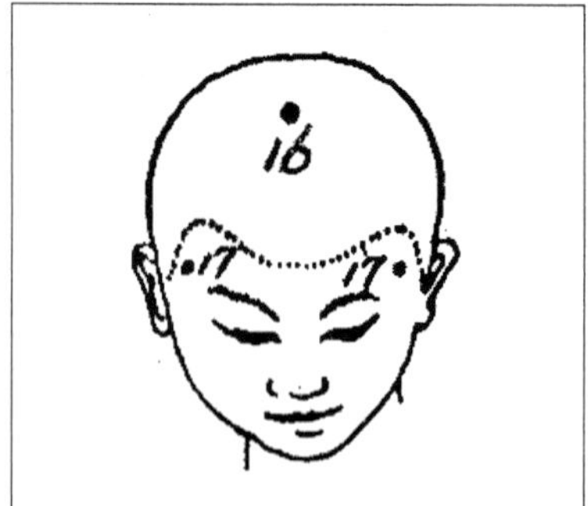

16. BAIHUI ("HUNDRED CONVERGENCES")

Located on the Du meridian, the Baihui point is found by tracing with your thumb and forefingers from the tops of your ears ascending upwards to the top of the head. Meeting at the top in the center, and moving slightly back. This point mostly points upward to the sky and receives Yang energy. Careful and correct stimulation of this point can relieve headaches, dizziness, sleeplessness, and high blood pressure.

17. TAIYANG

Located on the head in the temporal region within the superficial parameters of the Upward Dantian, the Taiyang point is an unusual point that is not located on any channel or meridian. This extra point is often referred to as Extra point number 2. The Taiyang points are located on both sides of the head. Careful and correct stimulation of this special point can relieve migraine, common cold, eye diseases and palsy.

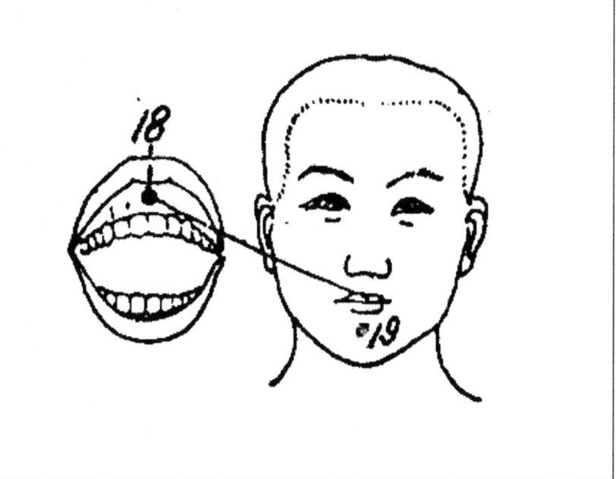

FIGURE D-4

18. YINJIAO

Located at the end of the Du meridian, the Yinjiao point is located on the frenulum of the upper lip (that part that connects the upper lip to the upper gum). Careful and correct stimulation at this point will relieve teeth and gum pain, cardiac pain, as well as to help correct jaundice.

19. CHENGJIANG ("SALIVA RECEIVER")

Located at the end of the Ren meridian, the Chengjiang point is located below the bottom lip and the top of the chin. Careful and correct stimulation at this point can relieve teeth and gum pain, facial paralysis, excessive salivation, as well as relieve canker sores.

20. YONGQUAN ("GUSHING SPRING")

Located on the Kidney channel, the Yongquan (known as the

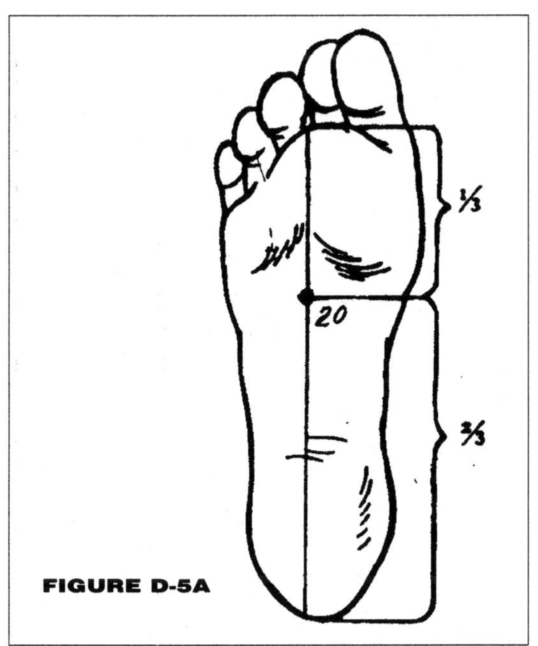

FIGURE D-5A

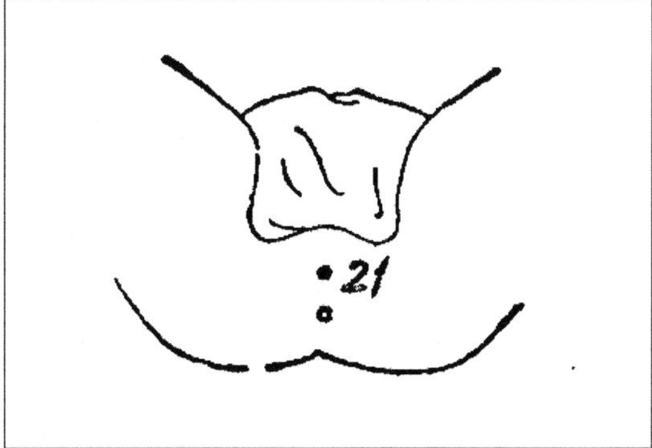

FIGURE D-5B

"Gushing or Pouring Spring," or sometimes "Bubbling Well") point is found by drawing a vertical line from between the second and third toes through the center of the sole of the foot to the heel. Then, measure 1/3 of the way down from the top of the foot, and mark a horizontal line across. Where the two lines intersect is the precise Yongquan point. It is usually found near the center of the ball of the foot on both feet. Careful and correct stimulation of this point is good for correcting high blood pressure, relieving insomnia, and headache.

21. HUIYING ("YIN CONVERGENCE")

Located on the Ren Meridian, the Huiying point is located between the scrotum/vagina and the anus. Careful and correct stimulation of this point can help correct irregular monthly periods, provide relief from hemorrhoids, relieve respiratory failure, and involuntary seminal emission.

CHAPTER THREE

CIRCUMSTANCES FOR OPTIMUM PRACTICE

TIME OF PRACTICE

In the traditional practice the times of the day of the day are considered very important. In other words it takes 24 hours to complete a rotation of the Earth. Therefore, the tradition holds that it takes twenty four hours to complete the internal energy's flow throughout the twelve channels. In other words, every two hours one channel is more emphasized in the internal flow of energy. The traditional "Chi" clock is as follows:

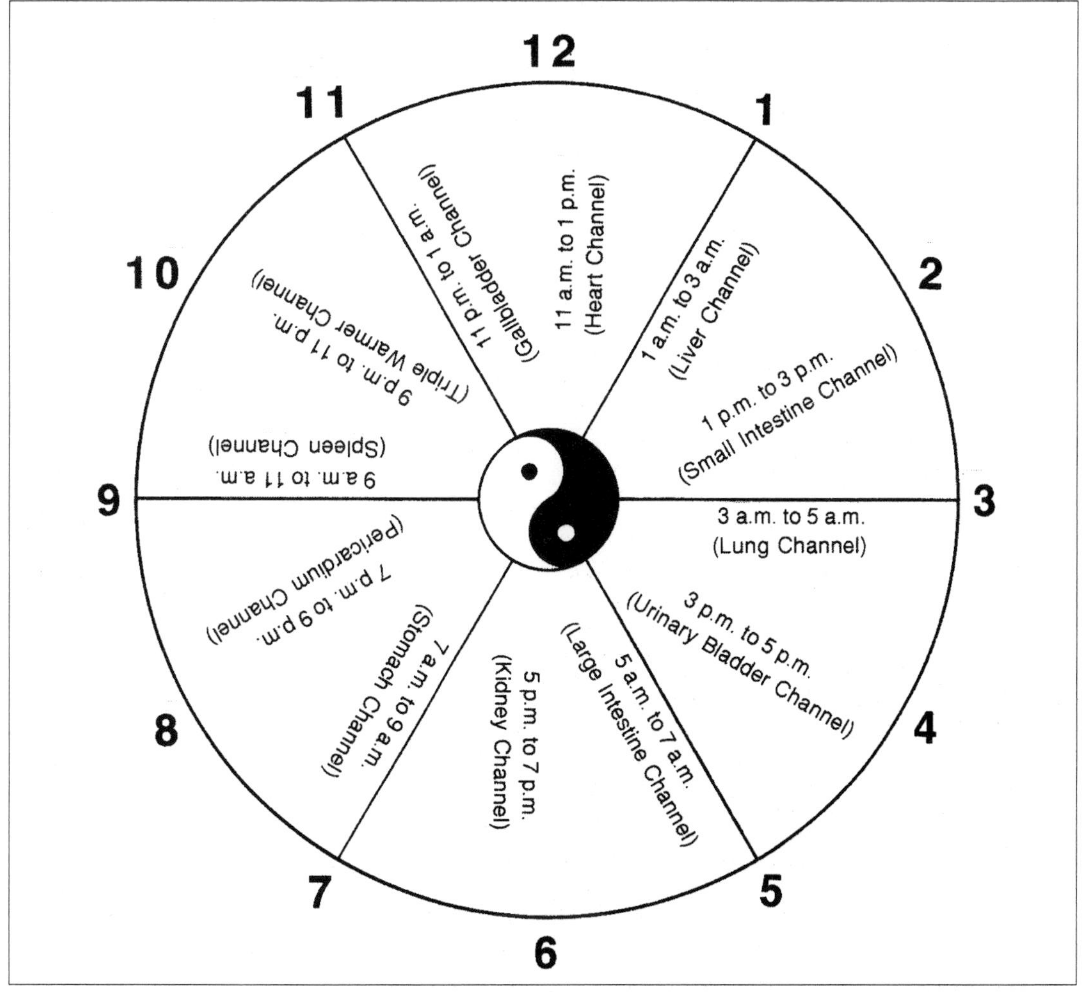

TIME OF DAY CHANNEL		
11 p.m. to 1 a.m. (Gall Bladder Channel)	7 a.m. to 9 a.m. (Stomach Channel)	3 p.m. to 5 p.m. (Urinary Bladder Channel)
1 a.m. to 3 a.m. (Liver Channel)	9 a.m. to 11 a.m (Spleen Channel)	5 p.m. to 7 p.m (Kidney Channel)
3 a.m. to 5 a.m. (Lung Channel)	11 a.m. to 1 p.m. (Heart Channel)	7 p.m. to 9 p.m. (Pericardium Channel)
5 a.m. to 7 a.m. (Large Intestine Channel)	1 p.m. to 3 p.m. (Small Intestine Channel)	9 p.m. to 11 p.m. (Triple Warmer Channel)

The seasons Spring and Summer are more Yang, so effective practice would be generally balanced with Yin organ practice time. Autumn and Winter belong to Yin, so Yang organ practice time is preferred. For example, the time of 3 a.m. to 5 a.m. is generally a good time to practice in the Spring. This time is the lung's time which is one of the solid (Yin) organs, and therefore most optimal for achieving balance with the season. Likewise, 5 a.m. to 7 a.m. is generally a good time to practice in Autumn, because this is considered the large intestine's time. The large intestine is one of the six hollow (Yang) organs.

Of course, because of job constraints and personal reasons, we are often times unable to follow the "Chi" clock. Therefore, it is best to try and exercise early in the morning, when your particular area of the Earth is less polluted, the air more fresh, the Sun is just coming up, and prior to when local traffic begins to peek. In this way, your practice benefits from the "modern world's" most optimal conditions.

PLACE OF PRACTICE

The most optimal place to practice is in or near a forest (pine or cypress). Avoid sweet scented trees, such as Oleanders. As the energy and smell is not good to absorb through air or energy. However, most trees give off good Chi and oxygen, and absorb negative energy and pollution.

Surprisingly or not, trees have their own Lower Dantian. It's not unusual to see Chi Kung practitioners communing with trees, exchanging what's good for the other, and yes looking about or trying to find the trees Lower Dantian. As in humans, there is usually an identifying knot, which may look very like the Shenque(or, navel) point. Sensing about below this point, by touch or by utilizing the hands like a magnet may help to locate the tree's Lower Dantian which is considered the tree's power center much like a human's.

Ideally a place that has an abundance of trees, small hills, and water is usually a place where the air is fresh and a good place to practice Chi Kung. Again we don't always have the greatest locale, or the most ideal place. However, areas that are near factories that release harmful pollutants or excessive car exhaust are to be avoided if at all possible. Practice in the cleanest environment nearest to you, or practice indoors.

Scorching hot sunny afternoons ought to be avoided. Rainy days, fog, and extremely windy conditions should be avoided as well. Practicing outdoors during rainy and foggy conditions can infect the lungs with excess moisture, and causes stagnate Chi to build up in the lungs and in the channels. Practicing, under these extreme conditions, is better done indoors with the window slightly opened.

PERSONAL CONSIDERATIONS

Emptying the stomach before Chi Kung practice, or practicing just after eating a hearty meal should be avoided. During Chi Kung practice the energy in the stomach and intestines is more active, and having the proper amount of nutrition in the digestive tract is more productive. Therefore, fasting or over eating should be avoided prior to Chi Kung practice. In the tradition the rule is: "Hunger harms the Chi, while to be gorged harms the stomach." Wait at least a half an hour after a meal before engaging in Chi Kung practice.

The clothes should be comfortable and loose fitting. Do not wear tight belts, clothing, high heeled or uncomfortable shoes while practicing. Concerning shoes, barefoot on fresh, soft grassy covered ground is the best.

Try to take care of relieving waste from the body prior to practicing. Otherwise, practicing while your kidneys or bladder are under such strain may cause severe problems in the body's ability to relieve itself properly.

It's advisable for women while menstruating to halt practice for a few days. For practice under these conditions may cause an increase in the blood flow. On the other hand, practice is advisable if you have trouble bleeding (extravasated), if the bleeding is too less, or cramping (dysmenorrhoea) is occurring. However, don't become too tired while practicing. Rest as needed.

Finally, don't be in a hurry to learn Chi Kung. You cannot in one day learn all there is about the practice. It takes time to increase your internal strength and harmonize your system with the internal chi, as well as the external chi (or, the environment). You won't make any discoveries by trying too hard. Listen to others who may say something that will help you understand the practice more. Take your time. Enjoy the process of learning.

In time you will learn more then you can imagine, so employ patience. In patience you will come to appreciate the texture and fibers of yourself and the personal rewards Chi Kung practice and it's discipline will bring.

CHI KUNG'S UNIQUE EFFECTS

Chi Kung practice can lead one ultimately into a state of protective inhibition, so be careful to avoid falling asleep when practicing. Protective inhibition requires you to be an alert, as well as relaxed state. So, don't be alarmed if you find yourself slipping into a deeply relaxed state when practicing.

Correct Chi Kung practice will make the practitioner more alert. Chi Kung practice helps systematize the electric activity of the brain cells of the cerebral cortex to increase brain functions. In other words, the more relaxed you are, the easier it is to focus, and the more you are capable of experiencing the blending of external and internal energies.

After exercise the practitioner will feel calm and relaxed, instead of out of breath as in some forms of exercise. You may sweat more as you continue to practice over a period of years. This is natural, and is no cause for alarm. This usually means that toxins that inhibit the bodies functions are able to secreted without any inhibition.

Essentially what happens when you practice Chi Kung is that at some point in the practice, usually at the beginning, the channels and meridians are dredged and the bad energy or inhibitions come out or are removed. This dredging process may seem uncomfortable. At times the process may seem tiring or somewhat painful. It is in times like this that you need to be careful to be following the correct form and principles. After some time, you may find yourself sweating less, and feeling great amounts of energy at your command when you finish practicing.

The chi and the blood are harmonized throughout the system as you practice and develop stronger internal energy to throw out the weaker, irregular, or bad chi. Ultimately by the time you have completed practicing the form and you are at the final stage of the particular form's practice and are receiving and storing chi, the chi and blood are harmonized and a reserve of energy is stored in the Lower Dantian to ward off stress and disease.

At this level of practice, sweating may occur again at various stages of practice. However, this could be a continuous dredging still occurring; new channels, meridians or points opening; or, an excess of bad chi (toxins) being eliminated. Profuse sweating with a feeling of dizziness during practice can be a sign of weakness, or that the flow of Chi is being hindered or not flowing properly.

Looking at the hands is a great indicator in determining the effectiveness of the flow of Chi. Sometimes beginners have cold, white hands that lack clear definition of the chi and blood's circulation. The ends of the fingers are sometimes shriveled, and the nails brittle. The nails may lack any definite pink, red, or further definition in the cuticles. These indications in the hands or feelings of cold in the body, indicate that the chi's circulation is likely incomplete in all twelve channels; or, that the chi and the blood are failing to harmonize properly.

Correct practice performed regularly and over a period of time will usually change the appearance of the hands. Moreover, the hands (as well as the feet) will not always be so cold. The ends of the fingers will fill out more, becoming round, and less shriveled. The nails will become stronger, the color of the nails will become more red and pink, and the cuticles more defined. The Chi and blood flow will be in harmony, and a gradual, continuous subtle feeling of warmth and energy while practicing will occur.

Often when Chi Kung practitioners finish practicing any form of Chi Kung exercise, there hands are still warm and tingling. Closer inspection of the palms reveals visually a variety of red and white spots. The red spots are thought of as blood, and the white spots thought of as Chi. Along the same lines, over a period of many years of Chi Kung practice, a white circle may form around and encompass the Laogong point in the center of the palm. This means that the Laogong point has opened up more and is able to emit and receive more chi to and fro any direction.

DIRECTION OF PRACTICE

Chi Kung practice is more favorable when the direction your body faces is considered. The back of your body is considered Yang and is tonifying. The front of the body is Yin and is purging. The direction the back of the body faces is important for absorption of certain elements lacking. The direction the front faces is important when wanting to purge, needing a certain element to help purge, or to avoid facing a certain direction in which the body is in excess of a certain element.

In the traditional Chi Kung practice the five elements are employed to discern the direction most beneficial for practice (Figure 43). However, for the average practitioner with no outstanding problems, the south is optimal where fire energy can be utilized to purge built up stresses, and energize the spirit in practice. While the back faces North and receives Water energy to tonify the kidneys.

CHAPTER FOUR:

THE FIVE ELEMENTS

THE FIVE ELEMENTS CYCLE

The five elements have an endless cyclical relationship with each other: Metal generates water, water generates wood, wood generates fire, fire generates earth, earth generates metal, and so on again and again. These elements often oppose, conquer, or interact with each other. For instance, metal conquers wood, wood defines the earth, earth restricts water, water diffuses fire, fire shapes metal.

The five elements can serve as a blueprint for everyday living. Providing a variety of aspects both in people's lives and nature. In the human, the elements take on characteristics through the vital organs, energy, channels, the senses, physical characteristics, and emotions. In nature, they share aspects with flavors, colors, conditions, directions, and seasons.

For instance, anger and yelling should be avoided if it all possible. Yelling brings the Chi up, and causes the liver/gallbladder energy (wood) to be excessive in the system. Anger is an attribute of wood. Therefore, excessive anger could signify or lead to a liver or gallbladder problem. To counteract this, it is best to seek calm and avoid the excesses of anger. However, if anger wins or you are able to determine you have a liver or gallbladder problem, it is best

CHART 4-A
FIVE ELEMENTS (HUMAN)

ELEMENT	SOLID (YIN) ORGANS	HOLLOW (YANG) ORGANS	SENSE ORGAN	PHYSIQUE	EMOTION
WOOD	LIVER	GALL BLADDER	EYE	TENDON	ANGER
FIRE	HEART	SMALL INTESTINE	TONGUE	PULSE	JOY
EARTH	SPLEEN	STOMACH	MOUTH	MUSCLE	OVER THINKING
METAL	LUNG	INTESTINE	NOSE	HAIR/SKIN	SORROW
WATER	KIDNEY	BLADDER	EAR	BONES	FEAR

CHART 4-B

FIVE ELEMENTS (NATURE)

ELEMENT	COLOR	FLAVOR	CONDITION	DIRECTION	SEASON
WOOD	BLUE	SOUR	WIND	EAST	SPRING
FIRE	RED	BITTER	HEAT	SOUTH	SUMMER
EARTH	YELLOW	SWEET	WET	CENTER	SUMMER
METAL	WHITE	ACRID	DRY	WEST	AUTUMN
WATER	BLACK	SALTY	COLD	NORTH	WINTER

CHART 4-C

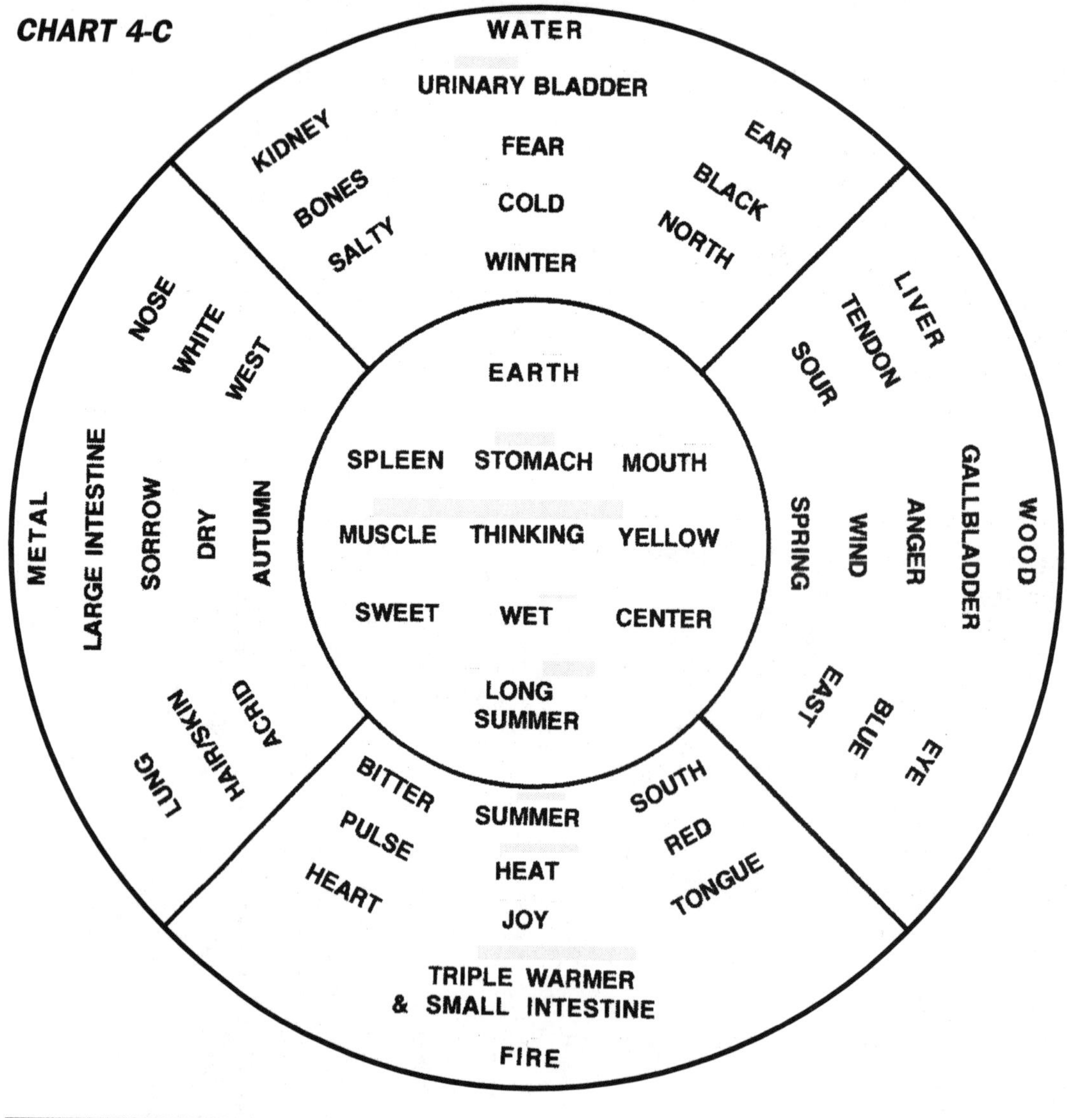

to seek calm and let your breath (lung energy/metal) be even and relaxed.

If you are excessively angry, your anger will ultimately lead to sorrow. This sorrow is natural as the body seeks to counteract excessive liver or gallbladder energy (anger). Sorrow is an attribute of metal (lung energy). Utilize this sorrow (lung/large intestine) energy to bring the anger under control. Other attributes of the lung/large intestine energy that will help to counteract the angry state would be to avoid using piercing eyes (the eyes are a sense organ attribute of the liver/gallbladder energy, or wood) to project your anger. Instead, concentrate on breathing gently through your nose (a sense organ attribute of the metal element or lung or large intestine energy) as if smelling a flower.

If you become overly sad (metal), then counteract your sadness with joy and be free of your sadness. Joy is an attribute of fire (heart/triple warmer/small intestine energy). Excessive sadness will ultimately lead to joy. Use the tongue to gently touch your upper teeth ridge to join your Du and Ren meridians, and circulate your chi on the small orbit. Thereby creating the Pulmonary circulation previously discussed. This practice will help to achieve joy and overcome your sadness.

Excessive joy can drain on the heart; as well as the triple warmer and small intestine energies. Very likely excessive joy signifies a heart/triple warmer/or small intestine energy obstruction. Utilize the water/kidney energy which may appear as fear to come into play to put out the excessive fire/heart energy.

However, don't confuse happiness and joy with positive energy. Happiness and joy in excess manifests in an overly excited person. Excited perhaps about a person they just met who they feel is "great", yet they've only known this particular person a relatively short time.

It is useful to increase the kidney energy to combat the heart related energy problem. Therefore, listen more (the ear is a sense attribute of the water/kidney energy) to those around you, and be less apt to jump into situations with loud jubilation and excitement. Excitement that will continue to fuel the untamed heart and lead to more problems.

Excessive fear may signify a troubled kidney or urinary bladder or an over stimulation of these energies. Excessive will likely lead to reason. Logically, the person attempts come to a conclusion that their excessive fear is often not well founded and a waste of energy.

Calm fear by inhaling gently through the nose and exhaling

through the mouth as if blowing on a flute, and think clearly. Thinking is an attribute of earth (spleen and stomach energy). The use of the stomach/spleen energy is useful to conquer fear and harness fear to your advantage.

However, over thinking can be problem and may very likely signify a spleen or stomach energy related problem. Over thinking can be controlled by keeping the Chi down. Often this may take the form of telling oneself to stop thinking even sometimes by activating anger (liver or gallbladder energy-organs related to wood); in order to quiet the voices in the head.

Utilize the eyes (a sense organ attribute of wood) to focus your thoughts or empty your mind, and concentrate the chi into the lower dantian to combat over thinking.

So in the preceding example, the circling of the five elements is complete, and continual. They can be used to conquer excesses. The example of utilizing the various sense organ attributes that correspond to the elements may or may not work for you at various times. So, utilize other attributes that correspond to the elements such as colors, flavors, directions, and attributes as they relate to the physique. The various aspects are useful in a variety of situations. Again the more naturally and simply they are applied, the more practical and useful the application of the attributes will be.

However, the best way to deal with emotions and problems if at all possible is to avoid extremes, and realize that all forms of emotions carried to excess drain the body of it's vital energy and lead to an overstimulation of the various organ's energies. Likely leading to an upset or disease of the system.

Ideally, it is best to just accept the various emotions and allow them to manifest in ourselves and others. Never carrying anything to excess.

Concerning Chi Kung form's practice or the self directed method, it is best to avoid practicing under emotionally extreme conditions. For example, if you are angry and you practice, you very likely will increase your anger and hurt an already ailing liver or gallbladder. Likewise, if under the strain of any excessively emotional state it is best to sit quietly and apply the five elements, and bring yourself out the overly emotional state before practicing Chi Kung.

Always try to avoid extremes and seek moderation. Control and come to know yourself. After you come to really know yourself, avoid judging others. Be easy on yourself, and avoid overindulgence in food, sex, recreation and in seeking pleasure.

CHAPTER FIVE:

FOLLOWING NATURE'S PATH WITH THE WILD GOOSE

Practitioners of Wild Goose Chi Kung follow the day in the life of a wild goose as it wakes up to greet the sky, spreads it's wings, draws it's wings back, pats water and flies away, drinks water, flies up to the sky, looks for food, looks for the nest, sleeps peacefully, and wakes up to greet yet another day. These movements follow closely the movements of a wild goose in nature. The movements throughout the form are often alternated with moments of stillness.

How many times a day the Wild Goose Chi Kung should be practiced varies from individual to individual. Ideally for the most optimum results it is best to practice the form two to three times daily. The 64 forms can be practiced in their entirety in about 10-15 minutes. The 64 forms can be practiced all together, or various sequences can be taken out of context.

When you have a cold or a fever take rest and don't practice. Wait until the cold or fever passes through resting, then resume practice little by little. If you sense a cold coming on it's all right to practice, and see if by the time you finish practicing you feel the cold come out in your feet (Yongquan point) and hands (Laogong point). Shortly after such a reaction you may feel warmth and experience some sweating.

If the cold and flu persists after such a reaction, the cold or flu may progress. However, it won't be a drain, as it would have been had you done nothing in the early stages.

The method of Wild Goose Chi Kung is strong for eliminating and strengthening the system. Don't force the movements, to fit the form's requirements. Don't concentrate on the idea of power while practicing. The Wild Goose Chi Kung is most beneficial in developing power through the most subtle emphasis in movements, while holding no extreme tightness in the joints of the limbs or muscles.

Various types of Chi Kung prescriptions or pithy formulas for counteracting trouble or disease can be complicated and specific. Any deviation from the prescription or pithy formula can cause more trouble than good. Wild Goose Chi Kung practice offers a more holistic approach encompassing a variety of postures tied together like a chain. Meant to be practiced to address the entire system; as well as, the whole person.

It's all right if mistakes are made in Wild Goose Chi Kung practice. No harm will come to the practitioner, as long as they decrease the mind's emphasis on chi flow, and allow the natural laws of motion to move the body and the chi.

This is the beauty of the Wild Goose Chi Kung which may be one of the safest form's of Chi Kung to practice, because the emphasis is more on employing the body's natural movements and tendencies to accomplish the form's requirements and to circulate the chi. Furthermore, as the body and mind methods of the form are mastered, the focus on the mind and body are to be less and less emphasized.

In other words, once the movements are learned, the practitioner empties the mind and lets go of all inhibitions. The higher level practice then calls for utilizing nature's forces such as: gravity, centrifugal force, momentum, velocity, equal force and gentle unbalanced force such as: the rocking back and forth or side to side on the soles of the feet, moving right to move left, moving up to move down, etc. to carry forward the requirements of the form's practice.

For example, in the opening posture of Wild Goose Chi Kung called "Spread Wings," the practitioner is encouraged to set the form into motion with small movements such as a slight, gradual unbalanced force of movement forward onto the balls of the feet, while gradually and slightly raising the heels off the ground. Naturally creating a forward incline plane with the soles of the feet, while simultaneously allowing the movement of the upper limbs to flow upward.

Like centrifugal force this outward movement leads into the next movement. The weight is moved more into the balls of the feet, and the heels are gradually raised more to increase the degree of the incline plane created with the soles of the feet. Further extending this outward force, helping to bring the arms up and outward. Then creating momentum to bring the arms up and back to gently curve backward; the gaze to look slightly upward; and the turning of the palms up to face the sky. All these movements set into motion by one small movement outwardly into the balls of the feet, that gained momentum and velocity and developed more motions of equal force.

The next movement that follows is called "Close Wings" wherein the torso gradually bends forward, bringing the upper limbs outward and downward. Ultimately, the palms (Laogong points) come inward to the Lower Dantian not by use of isolated force on the arms, hands or wrists. Rather, by following the movement of the weight to the backs of the heels, as the heels continue to be gradually lowered. Sensing and merging with the Earth's natural gravitational pull.

In essence, the more you allow the natural forces of motion such as centrifugal force, gravity, momentum, velocity, and angles of motion to be integrated gently and evenly in the practice, the more variables you will create for the softest and most gentle of movements. This, of course, will encourage the chi to flow more evenly and smoothly in your practice, and encourage the whole system to be apart of your practice. Ultimately if you can harmonize your internal and external movements with the universal laws of motion and gravity that exist externally and outside yourself, you will blend internal and external chi. By blending internal and external energies helps you to contact, receive, and circulate more chi from nature. This is one of the key essentials of Chi Kung practice.

The idea is to do the entire form with less force and to follow the natural laws of motion. By following the laws of motion, you are more likely to blend your movements with the nature around you, and actually achieve a state of harmony and flow with nature.

Hopefully as you correctly practice the form more you may come to understand more of how less and less is done, until non-action is achieved; and yet nothing is left undone or incomplete. The form becomes formless, yet there is still a form. More is done with less, because more of the whole is employed.

The earth rotates without isolated force. It is the interaction of centrifugal force (outward motion) and gravity (inward pull) that turns the Earth. The seasons and the other aspects of the five elements exist due to a whole process with and interaction with each other. Many forms of life have a purpose and a plan; a beginning, a middle, end, and rebirth. Just like the human's time span from birth until death and rebirth.

So the form of Wild Goose Chi Kung has structure, and applications for the flow of energy. Therein, defining a specific purpose and plan. A plan that carries that utilizes movements that employ nature and natural forces of motion. Not movements which are intended to be done in isolation. Rather, movements which are linked to each other like a complete chain. Movements that are continuous, and yet each link of the chain is important and clearly defined.

With the application of science and the laws of motion, the Wild Goose Chi Kung form in the traditional practice is to be mastered then forgotten. The mind is to be emptied, and the form allowed to follow nature's path. This is the traditional practice.

In this way, Wild Goose Chi Kung remains one of the safest forms of Chi Kung to practice. Very often it is the unclear or unfocused mind whose direction of chi may be the very cause of most problems that may occur if any from Chi Kung practice. However, it is the traditional approach of the Wild Goose Chi Kung that applies the natural laws of motion and dismisses the focus on the isolation of chi and the mental focus on the flow and direction of chi. Instead encouraging the flow of chi through natural movements, that make the possibility of flowing the chi "incorrectly" and causing any harm to decrease.

Since the Wild Goose Chi Kung's development in the Kunlun school of the Taoist branch of Chi Kung centuries ago, it remains a healthy, safe form of Chi Kung that will undoubtedly continue to promote enlightenment and health for many generations to come.

CHAPTER SIX:

BASIC MODEL OF HANDS AND STEPS USED IN WILD GOOSE CHI KUNG

Most systems, traditional and contemporary, have a basic model of hands and steps. Following the correct basics can help make the form easier to learn. Moreover, the basic model of hands and steps help make your practice more consistent, and create a strong foundation by which to train the body and mind. Furthermore, by following a precise basic structure in the hands and steps without always watching as you do it to see if you are doing it "right", is a useful way to train the Yi (or, mind) to master the basic steps.

After becoming better acquainted with the basic steps, check yourself occasionally to see if you are consistent and following the prescribed basic. The appearance of the basics will vary from person to person as each person's physique varies. In Wild Goose Chi Kung, following the correct basic is also useful for stimulating the proper points and channels necessary for proper chi flow. The basics and their applications as far as the flow of chi are as follows:

A. HANDS

1. PALM: The palm is relaxed. The wrist should also remain relaxed, (unless a particular posture calls for a flexing of the wrist) so the energy will not stop at the wrist and be unable to flow to the palm and fingers.

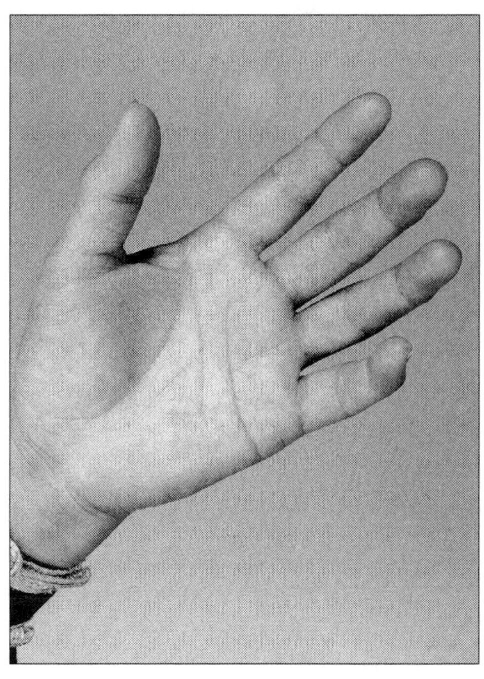

The five fingers are separated slightly, relaxed. Do not hold the thumb tightly. Maintain a roundness between the fore finger and thumb. In this way the Hegu point (located on the upper part of the hand in the fleshy portion between the thumb and forefinger) is opened. Furthermore, if the the area between the thumb and forefinger is rounded the Laogong point (located in the center of the palm, and straight through to the outside of the hand as well) is opened naturally as well.

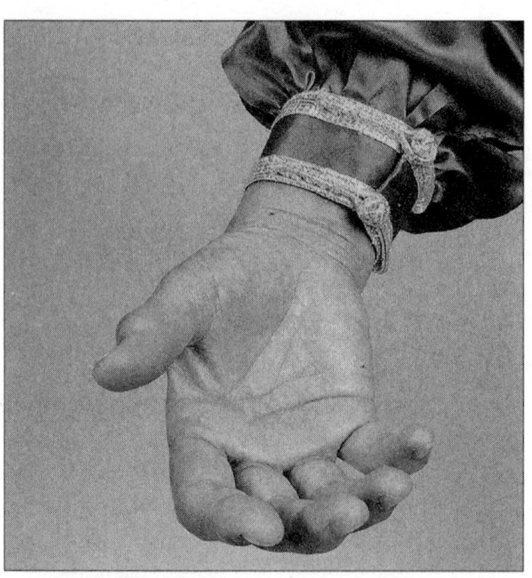

2. SCOOPING PALM: Curve the hand like a spoon, yet keep the fingers, palm, and wrist relaxed. This palm is used to "scoop up" fresh chi.

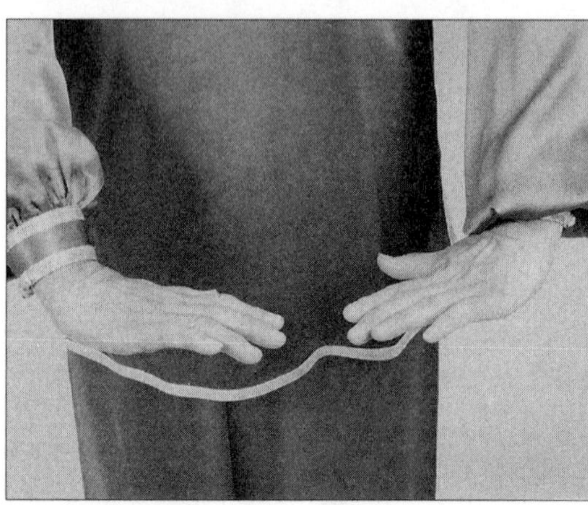

3. PRESSING PALM: The palms press downward, and fingers point towards each other. Then relax allowing the bad chi to be pulled out.

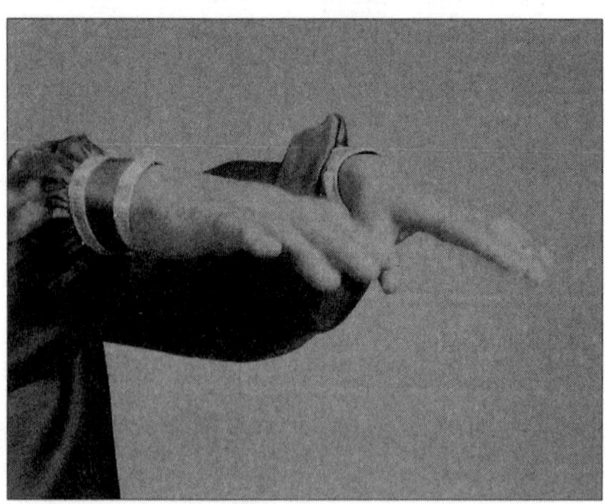

4. SHAKING PALMS: Utilizing the bridge of the palm (at the base of the fingers) vibrate the hand. Allowing the arms and fingers to vibrate as well. This active vibrating movement with the palms, vigorously stimulates the chi on the Yin and Yang channels on the hands and arms, and helps to dredge the channels and pull out bad chi.

5. RISING PALM: The rising palm helps bring Yang energy up.

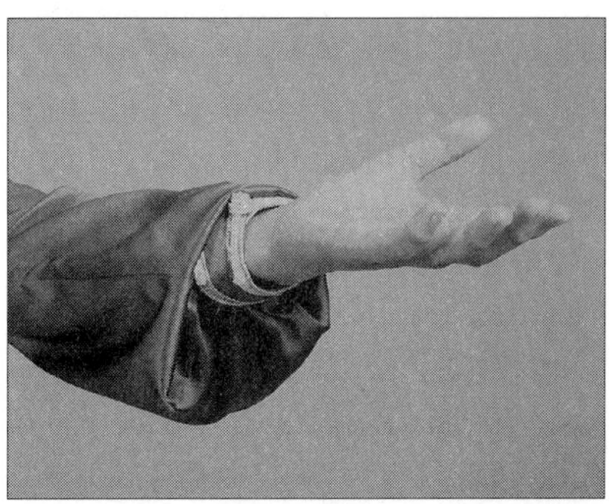

6. FALLING PALM: The falling palm helps bring Yin energy down.

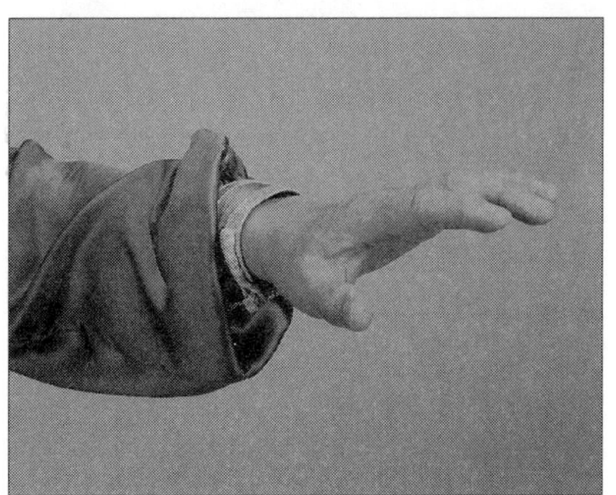

7. YIN PALM: The Yin palm faces inward and is erect and can store, circulate, or pull out chi.

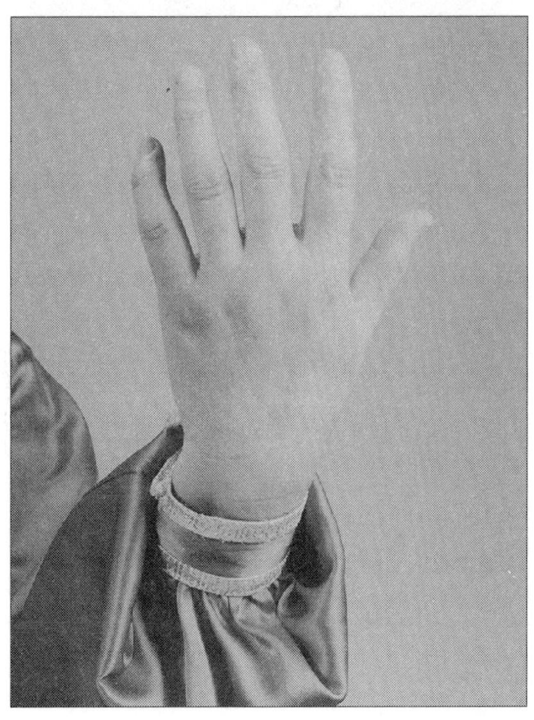

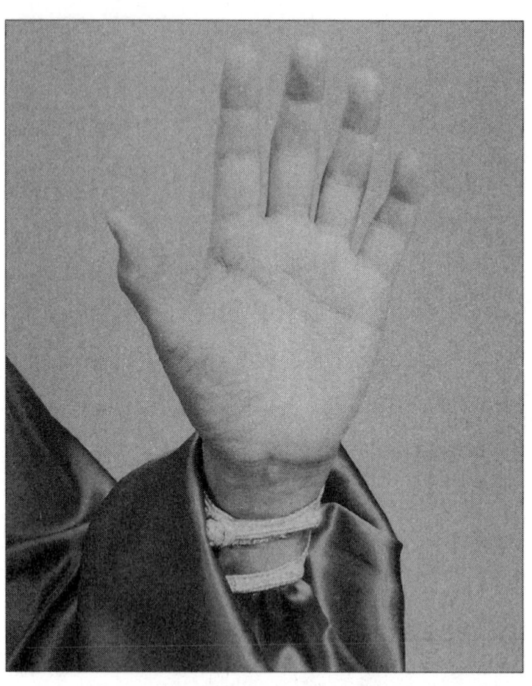

8. YANG PALM: The Yang palm faces outward and is erect and can contact, emit, or gather chi.

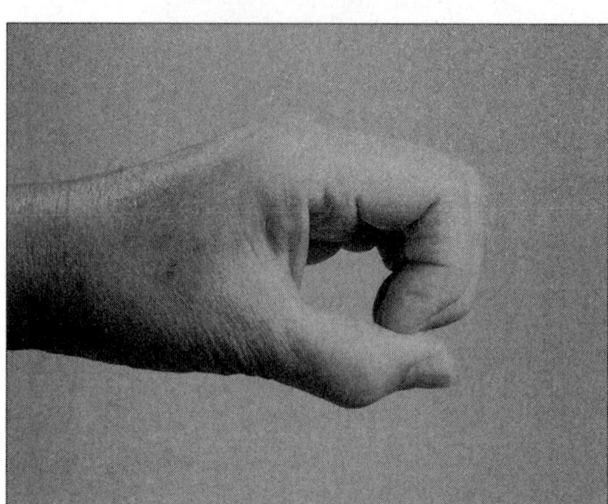

7. HOLLOW FIST: The Hollow Fist is made by curling the four fingers and placing the thumb over the fore and middle fingers to create a "hollow" fist. The Hollow Fist is used to store and pack chi.

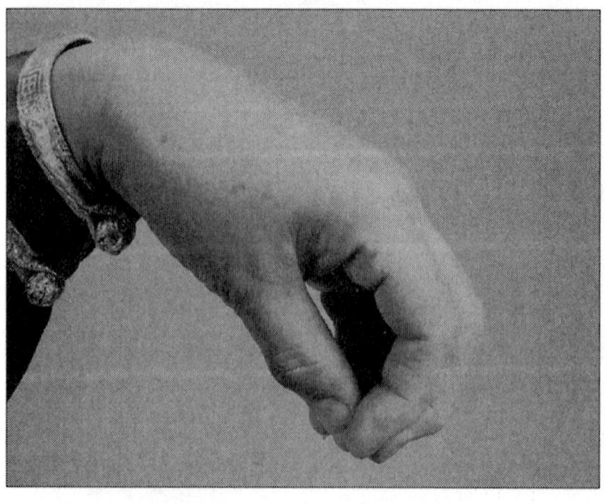

8 a. EAGLE'S BEAK: The Eagle's Beak is made by grasping the tip of the thumb with the tips of the four fingers, and relaxing the wrist and elbow. The Eagle's Beak can be used to store or pull out chi.

8 b.(ANOTHER ANGLE) Eagle's Beak. Here you can see the tips of the four fingers meet and gather together with the tip of the thumb.

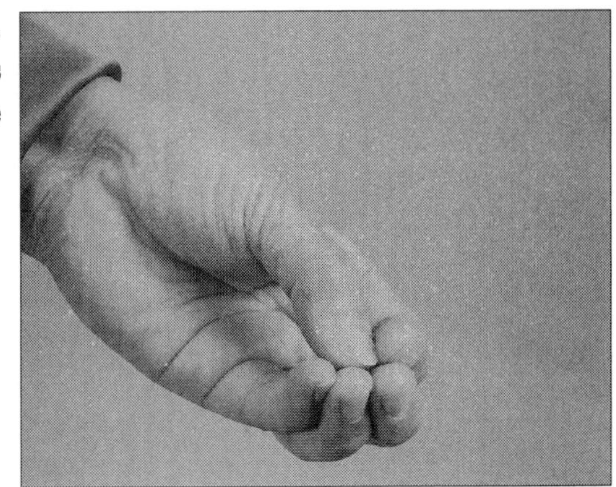

B. FEET

1 a. PARALLEL STANCE: The Parallel Stance is made by stepping out, maintaining a shoulder's width between the feet. Keeping the toes pointed straight forward, while maintaining the four characteristics of the parallel stance which are: Upright, straight, even, and steady.

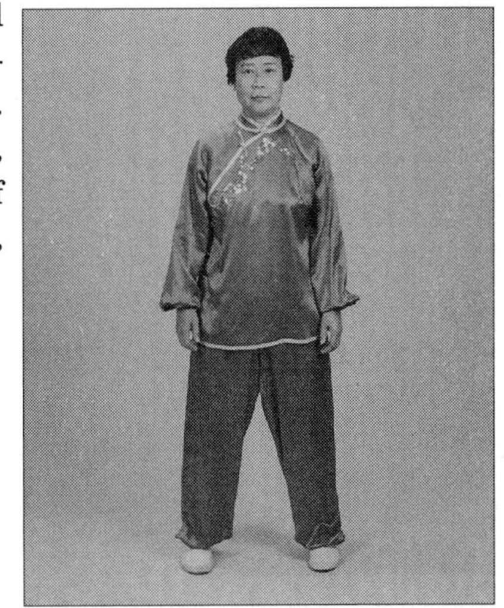

1 b. To check to see if your feet are shoulder width assume a stance, feet parallel, shoulder width, and then turn in the left heel on the ball to assume the same line as the right toe.

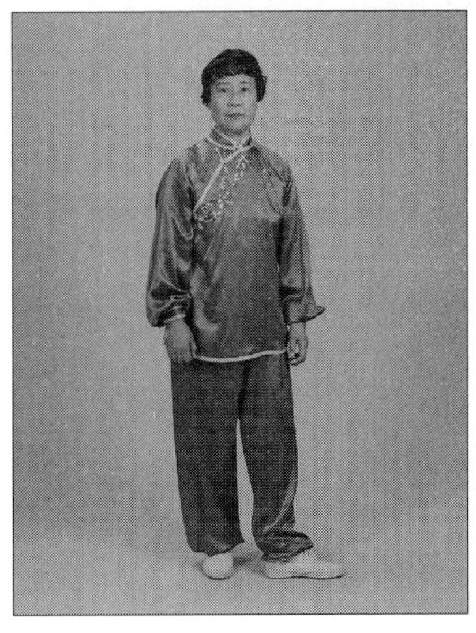

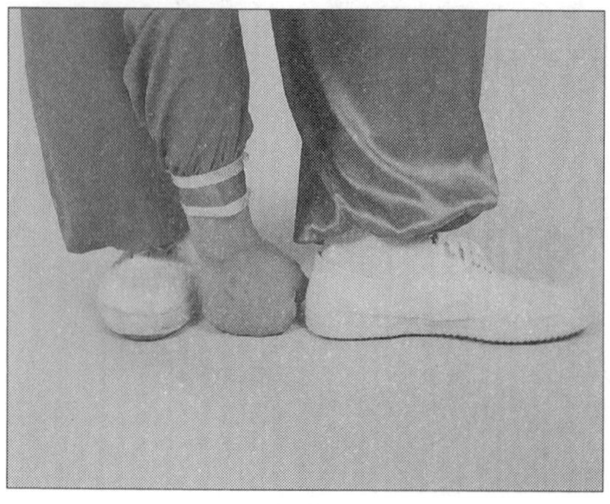

1 c. Then if you can place one fist between the space, your stance is your shoulder's width. Adjust accordingly.

Check your posture and stance quite often in the beginning of your studies, and after you have studied at great length periodically check to see if the toes are pointing precisely straight forward with the appropriate width. The purpose for the exactness is to encourage the balance of Yin and Yang by placing equal amount of pressure on the three Yin and Yang channels of the feet.

2. EMPTY STANCE: There are two empty stances in Wild Goose Chi Kung:

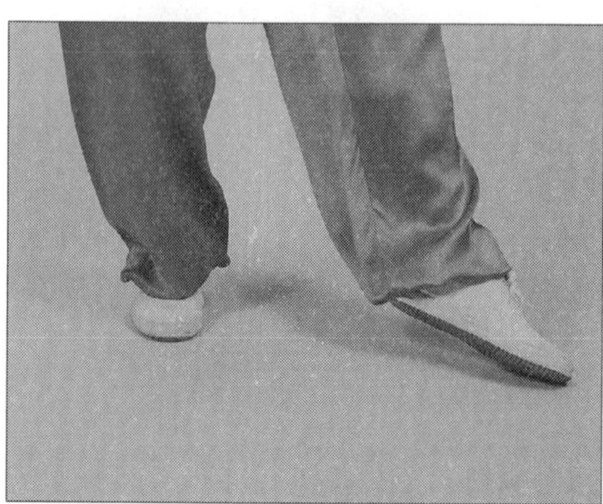

2 a.) Outer Edge of the Foot: In this stance the outer edge of the foot touches the ground lightly, and gradually weight is added with ensuing movements.

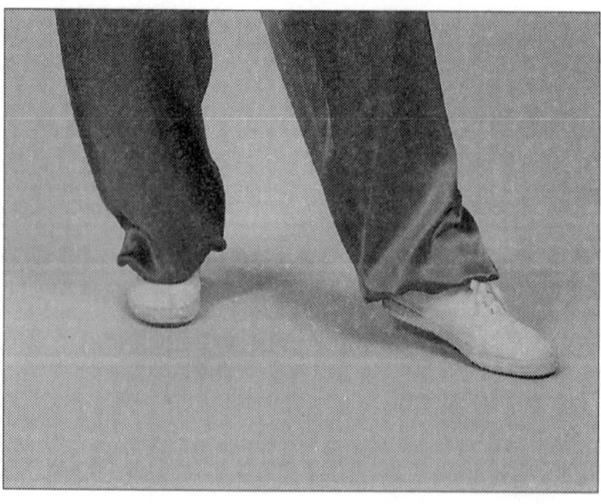

2 b.) Ball of the Foot: In this stance, the heel is raised and the ball of the foot rests on the ground. Keep the ankle relaxed, as the heel is slightly raised one to two of your fingers in height.

The purpose of both types of the Empty Stance is to open the Yongquan point (located near the center of the ball of the foot) of the empty foot, and contact the Earth's energy. Also to stimulate the channels on the feet.

3. RAISING AND DROPPING OF THE HEELS STANCE: There are two stances:

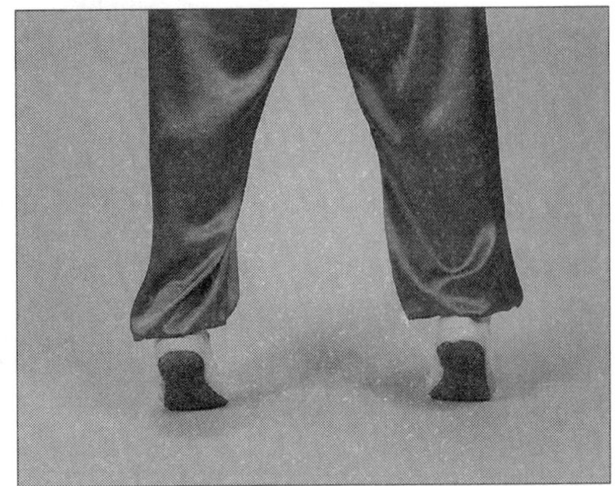

3 a.) Heels Up: Both heels raise up. In the parallel stance, as shown here, keep both the heels raised to the same height if possible. From an empty stance, moving the weight forward onto the balls of the feet, the back heel will raise higher because of the natural forward progression of the body's weight.

3 b.) Heels Down: There are two methods:

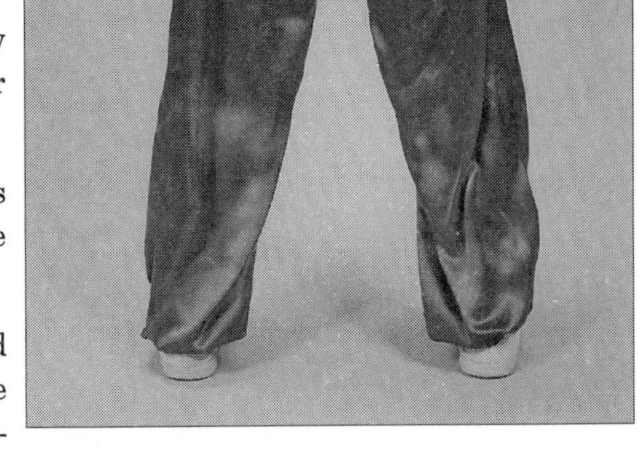

1. Relaxed: Lower the heels down slowly while coordinating the upper and lower limbs with the movement.

2. Force: Allow gravity to lower the heels suddenly. Sinking the body's weight into the rear heel or both heels.

The purpose of both the Heels Up and Heels Down step methods are to stimulate the energy on the three Yin and Yang channels of the feet, and help to move the limbs and the body without excessive force employed by the upper limbs or joints of the upper limbs.The Force/Heels Down method, creates a sudden shock that encourages the energy of the three Yin channels of the feet to come up, and the energy of the three Yang channels of the feet to come down to more effectively and strongly bring out bad chi.

CHAPTER SEVEN:

STEP BY STEP DETAILED INSTRUCTION OF WILD GOOSE CHI KUNG

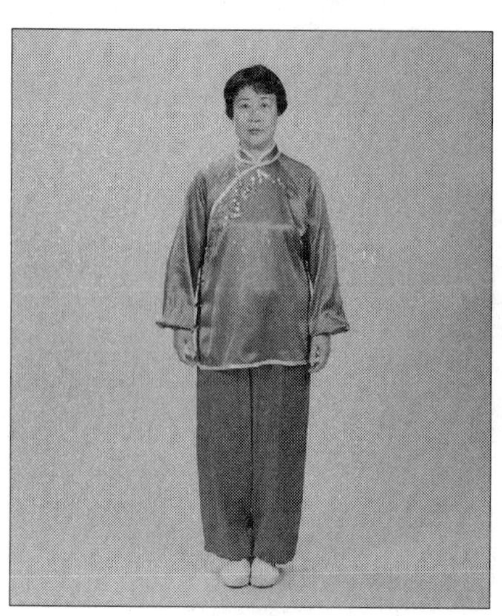

1. STARTING POSITION

1 a. Start with your feet together, toes pointing forward. Relax your whole body, don't hold your arms tightly at your sides. Close your mouth, and gently breathe through your nose. Rest the tip of your tongue gently on the back of the teeth ridge (Forward palate). Thereby, connecting the Du and Ren Meridians.

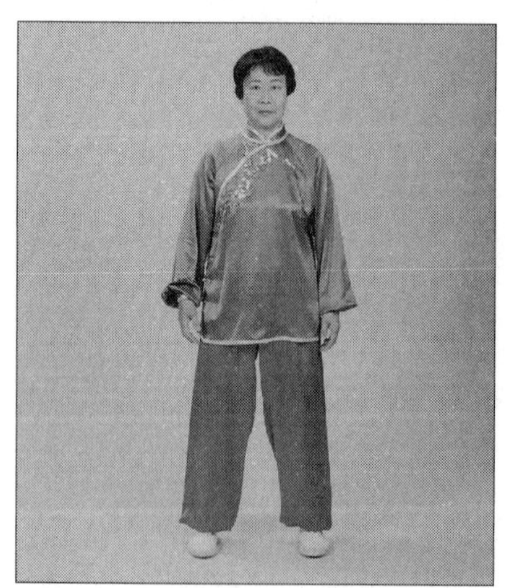

1 b. Take a step out to the left with your left foot, softly and gently by picking up the heel, ball of the foot, toe, and step out to the left a shoulder's width. Then place the left toe, ball of the foot, heel of the foot gently down in a parallel stance. Check to see if you are following the correct basic of a parallel stance (fist and one foot). Refer back to basic feet instruction: Parallel stance, if you need more explanation.

Imagine as if you were propping up something with your head. Keep your chin down slightly, and relax your shoulders and allow your arms to hang down naturally at your sides with the palms facing inward towards your thighs. The fingers are naturally separated, and the middle finger is line with the outer seem of your pants.

Relax your whole body, yet stand balanced and firm. Keep

your eyes open and your attention alert. Bring your Chi down to your lower dantian area. Empty your mind of all distractions, and stand quietly and calmly for awhile.

CHI ESSENTIALS: Taking the step out to the left and precisely assuming a Parallel stance without looking, trains the Yi (or, mind). Using the mind, with the eyes looking forward into the distance, maintains balance.When the tongue lightly touches the palate, saliva is likely developed. Don't spit out this health giving nectar. Rather, swallow to create more energy in the digestive tract. Remember, don't use force to touch the tongue to the palate.

Stand relaxed and achieve calmness. Receive the Chi at the top of the head at the Baihui point , and flow the Chi to the palms and feet. When the body is relaxed, circulate the Chi on the Du and Ren meridians promoting the Pulmonary Circulation (small orbit). Again don't use force or think too heavily about the tongue touching the palate. If the mouth is closed and you are gently breathing through the nose, your tongue is likely touching the palate naturally.

2. SPREAD WINGS

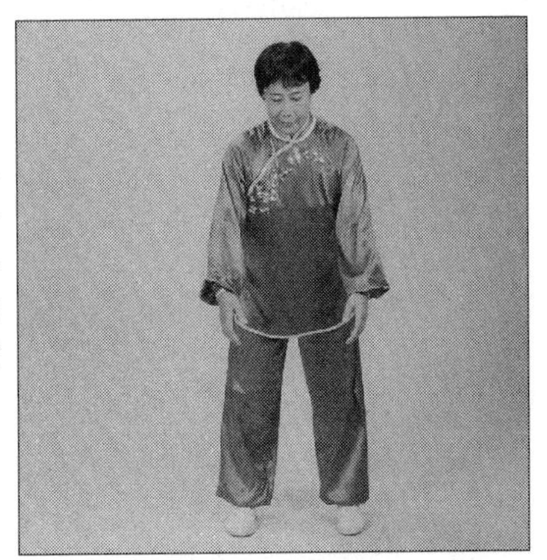

2 a. Raise both arms slowly to the front with the palms facing each other, while simultaneously allowing the weight to move forward into the balls of the feet. Let your focus stare slightly downward at the action of your hands.

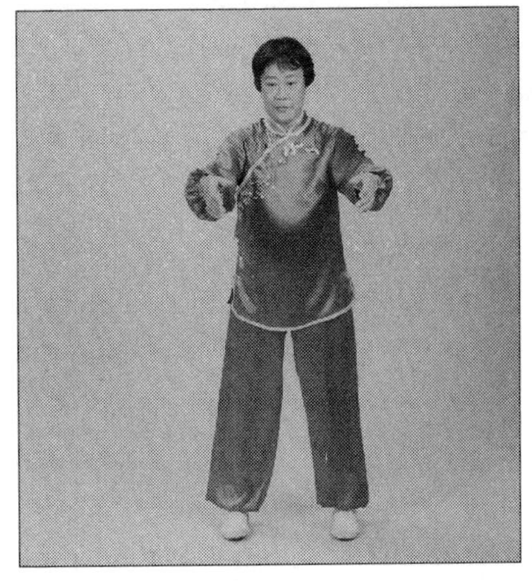

2 b. Continue to allow the arms to come up to shoulder level and turn out, while gradually moving the weight forward into the balls of the feet and gradually allowing the heels to come up.

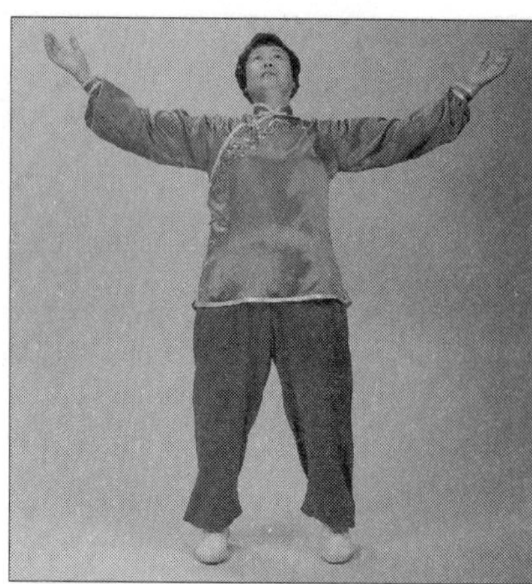

2 c-1. Gaze up at the sky (Yang) on an angle (not straight up), turning the palms to face upward to the sky, and the arms turn outward as if holding a huge ball. The heels should be fully off the ground by this point.

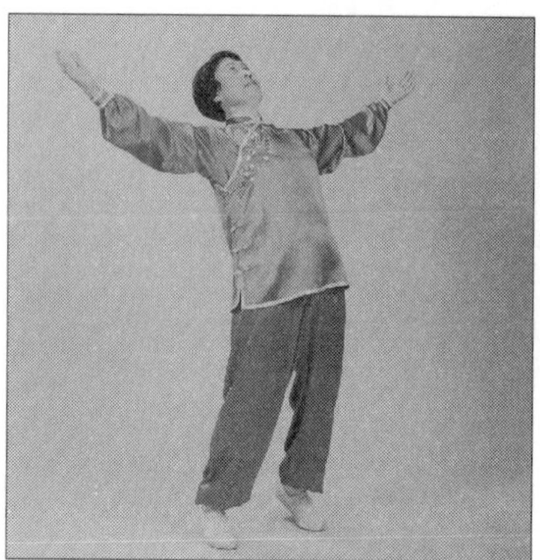

2 c-2. (ANOTHER ANGLE) Notice the head is not bent back so far that the Chi is hindered and unable to pass at the neck. The arms maintain a slight roundness, not locked out at the elbows which would hinder the free flow of chi. Finally notice the heels are off the ground, but the knees are not locked nor are they overly bent. Just relaxed slightly, gently encouraging the flow of Chi.

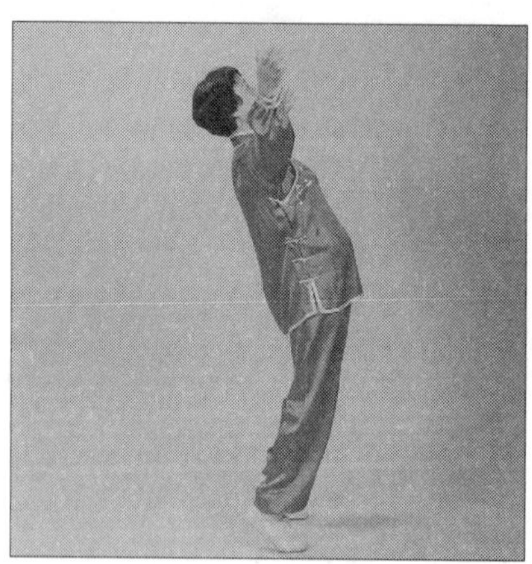

2 c-3. (ANOTHER ANGLE) Notice the natural curve from the top of the head, through the back, and down to the backs of the heels without any breaks at the joints where the chi would be stopped from flowing gently and naturally. Here you can also see the front of the body which is Yin faces up towards the Sky (Yang), and the back of the body which is Yang faces towards the Earth (Yin).

2 c-4. (REVERSE ANGLE) Here you can see the heels off the ground. If you can raise the heels more as you are going up, while moving the upper limbs upward then do so. If you can only raise them slightly, and maintain the natural curve from the top of the head through the backs of the heels then raise them only slightly. The important points are to hold no tightness in any of the joints, maintain the natural curve from the top of the head through to the backs of the heels, and encourage the soft, steady flow of chi in the posture.

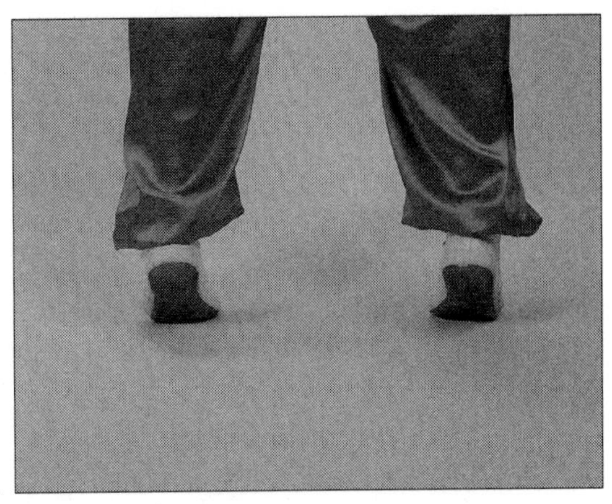

CHI ESSENTIALS: The raising of the hands upward in Spread Wings helps to open the 3 Yin channels on both hands. By turning the palms upward to the sky, the Laogong points on both hands are opened, and the Triple Warmer channel cleared. Receive Yang energy at the Laogong points as the palms face up to the sky. As Chi enters the Laogong points gently, then allow the Chi to pass through the Qihu point (The Qihu point opens easily, when the arms are spread open and apart.), and continue the flow of Chi down to the Lower Dantian. From there the Chi flows into the the Spleen and Stomach Channels. You may feel some warmth on both feet, as well on both hands and that's natural.

3. CLOSE WINGS

3 a. Gradually rotate the arms downward and inward, while the weight comes forward, and the torso gently straightens up. With the momentum created, the torso continues bending forward bringing the hands more downward and inward.

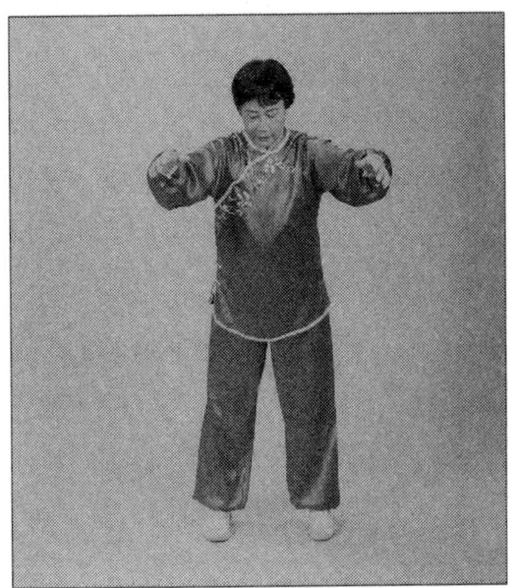

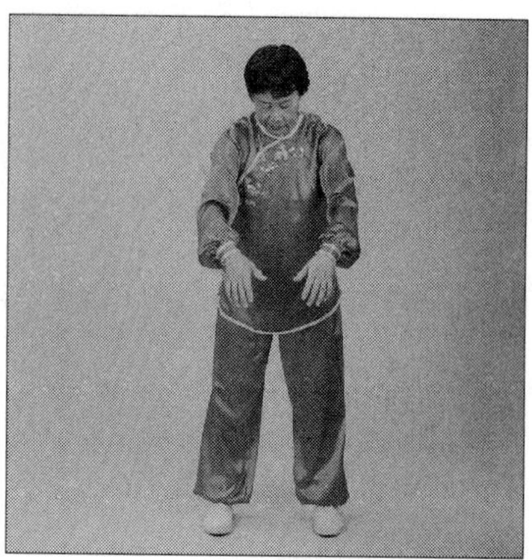

3 b. The palms continue traveling down to face the Lower Dantian. Make sure the hands are facing inward below stomach level with at least a ball's distance between the palms and the Lower Dantian.

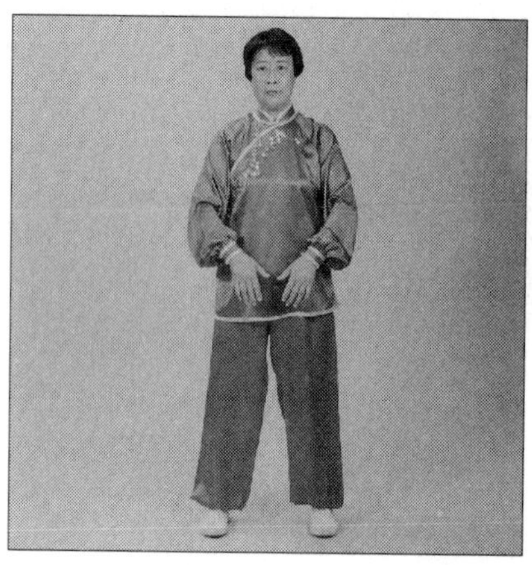

3 c. Then by allowing the heels to come down gently, this, in turn, helps bring the palms to come inward towards the Lower Dantian.

CHI ESSENTIALS: When the hands come down, guide the Chi into the Laogong point, and bring the Chi down to be stored in the Lower Dantian. By combining the forms Spread Wings and Close Wings, you are practicing to open and close the Lower Dantian; as well as training to move the Chi up and down.

The energy is contacted in the Lower Dantian before it moves on the first points of the Du, Ren and Chong Meridians. The Shenque point (Navel) is at the front, the Mingmen (Life Gate) is at the back, the Huiying is at the bottom, and the Baihui can be used as a direct energy gate from above to pass Chi down to the Lower Dantian. Furthermore, this form can be used to clear the upper, middle, and lower branches of the Triple Warmer.

The Lower Dantian is important because it connects the internal branches with the superficial branches of the body. Traditionally it is viewed as the storage place of Chi. Also, the place where semen is kept, or where the seed for another life is planted and nurtured.

4. DRAW WINGS TO THE BACK

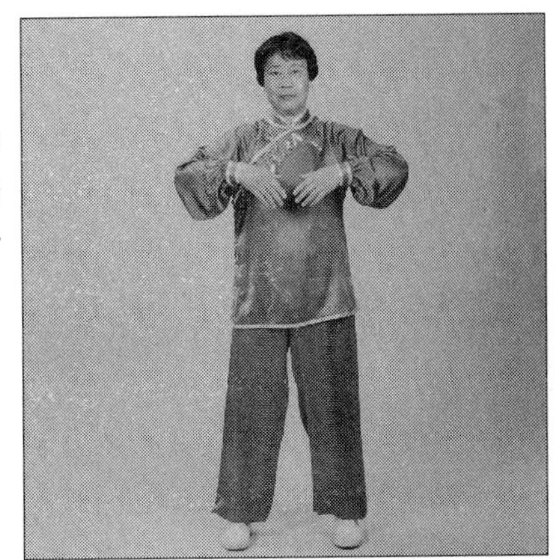

4 a. Lift the elbows, and raise both palms inward with the palms facing inward to the Middle Dantian, fingers naturally lay downward.

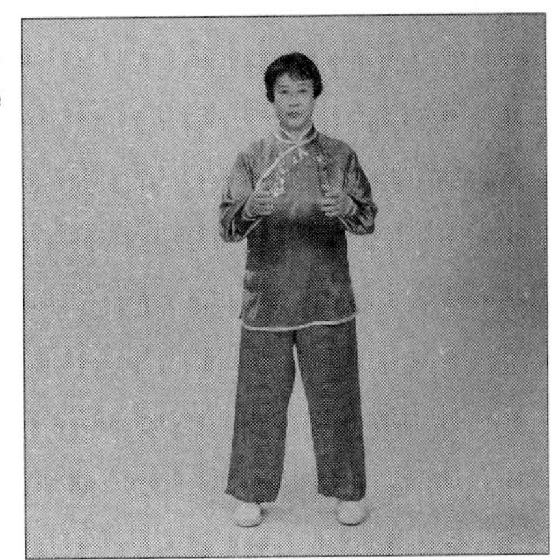

4 b. Consciously point the fingers forward, while gradually moving the weight into the balls of the feet.

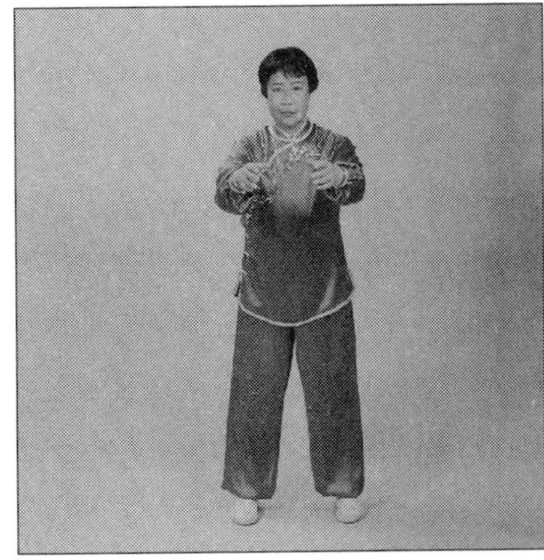

4 c. Continue gradually moving the weight forward into the balls of the feet, while gradually extending the arms straight forward out from the Middle Dantian.

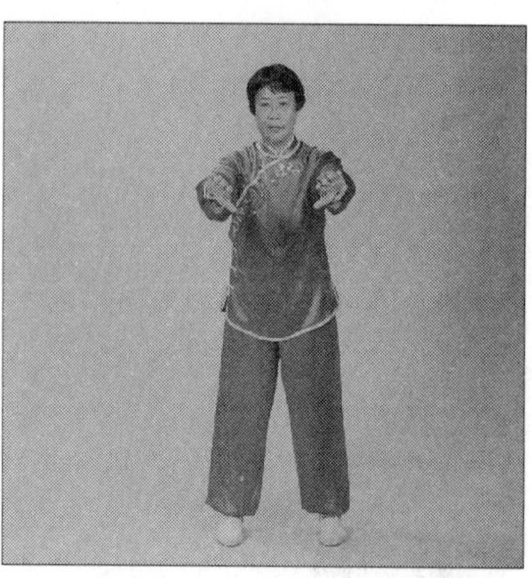

4 d. Then gradually raise the heels, while turning the palms outward.

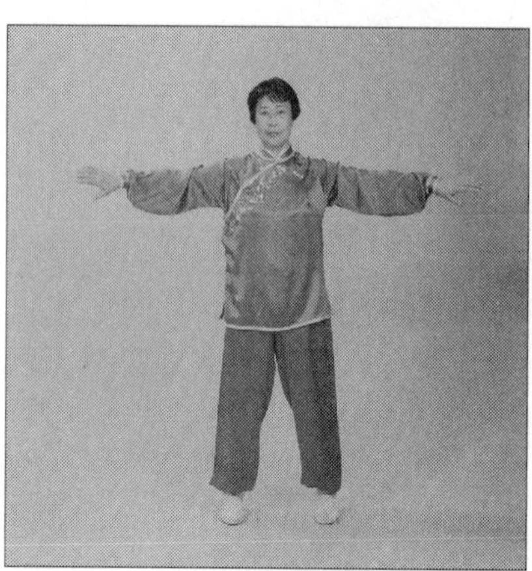

4 e. While continuing to gradually raise the heels, simultaneously rotate the arms to where the palms face back, and the arms come out to shoulder level.

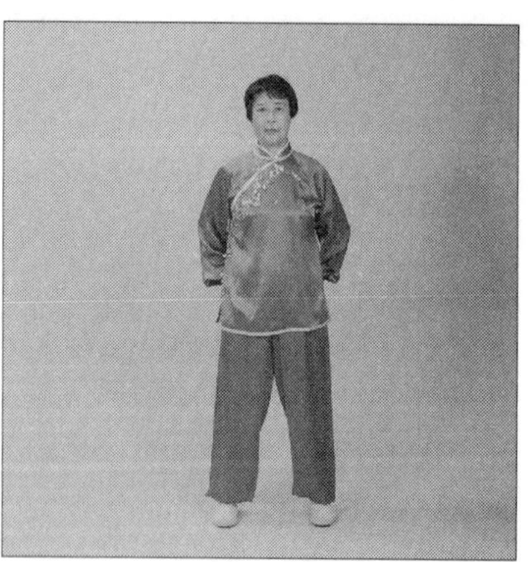

4 f. Then gently lower the heels to the ground, while simultaneously bringing the backs of the hands (the Hegu point) to rest on the buttocks (the Huantiao point).

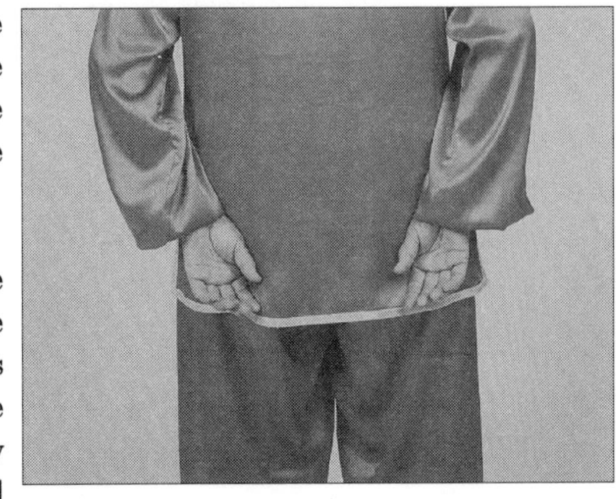

4 g. (REVERSE ANGLE/CLOSE UP) Here you can see the Hegu faces and rests on the Huantiao point. Notice the palms are relaxed, and not tightened or forced to make the points line up.

CHI ESSENTIALS: When raising the hands level with the breast bone store the Chi in the Middle Dantian. As the hands extend, the 3 Yin channels of the hands are stimulated. When the heels are gradually lifted, the Yongquan point is opened, and receive the Earth's energy (Yin). Pour fresh Chi from the Hegu point on the hand into the Huantiao point on the buttocks, when these two points contact each other. Thereby activating the Gall bladder channel. A warm sensation in the legs may follow, and this is natural.

5. JERK ARMS

5 a. Bend elbows and gently lift the backs of the hands up to the small of the back, while gradually raising the heels off the ground.

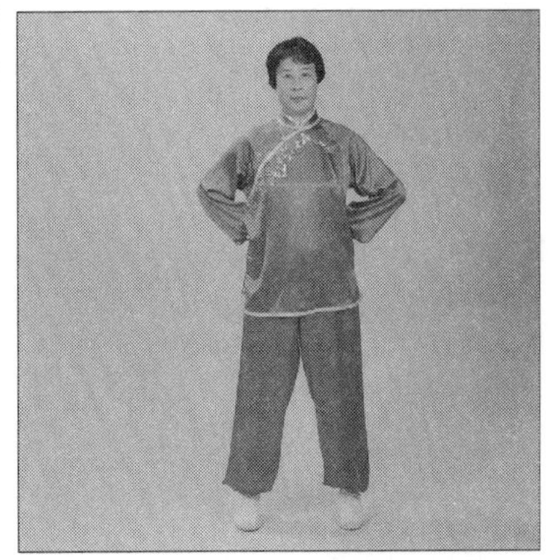

5 b. (REVERSE ANGLE/CLOSE UP) As you raise the hands to the small of the back, gradually transform your hands into Eagle's Beaks.

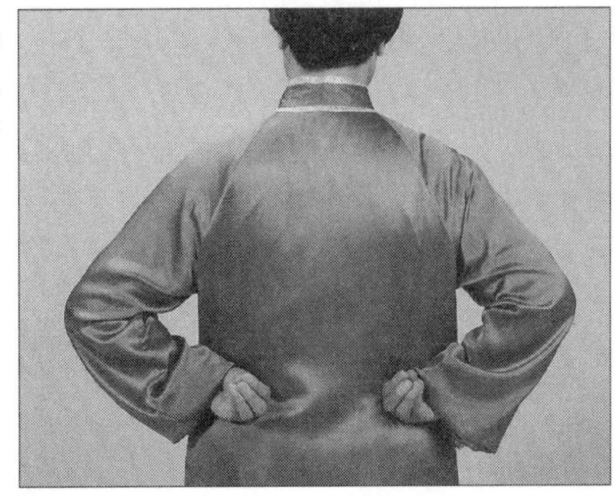

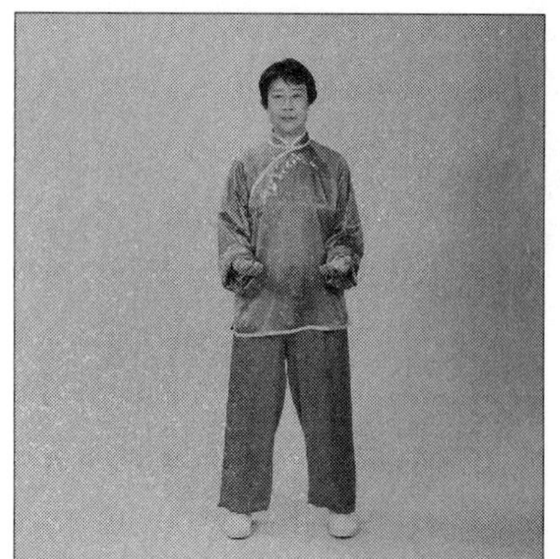

5 c. Then suddenly flick out the eagle's beaks and transform the claw hands back into palms. While suddenly dropping your heals to the ground (the force heels down method), and allowing your elbows to strike your sides. Palms face upward and slightly inward, while elbows are bent at a ninety degree angle. Look straight ahead, and stand balanced.

CHI ESSENTIALS: Remember that the Force/Heels Down method, creates a sudden shock that encourages the energy of the three Yin channels of the feet to come up, and the 3 Yang channels of the feet to come down to more effectively bring out bad Chi. In this form, the elbows simultaneously strike the sides of the waist, as both feet hit the ground to help drive the bad chi out through the hands and feet.

The palms remain facing upward with the elbows at the sides of the waist momentarily, in order to collect fresh Chi at the Laogong points on the palms of both hands.

6. DRAW WINGS TO THE BACK

Rotate the arms inward, and extend the arms forward, palms facing each other. Then repeat movements 4 c through 4 f.

CHI ESSENTIALS: See Chi Essentials for Form 4: Draw Wings To The Back.

7. JERK ARMS

Repeat movements 5 a through 5 c.

CHI ESSENTIALS: See Chi Essentials for Form 5: Jerk Arms.

8. LIFT ARMS

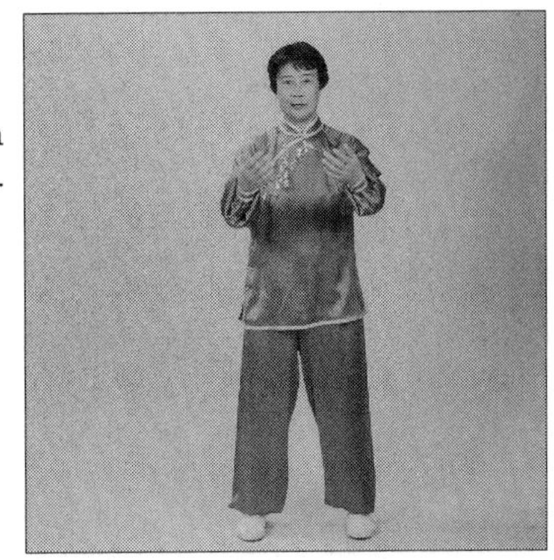

8 a. Slowly lift hands, palms forming Yin palms (or, facing inward) with fingers pointing slightly upward.

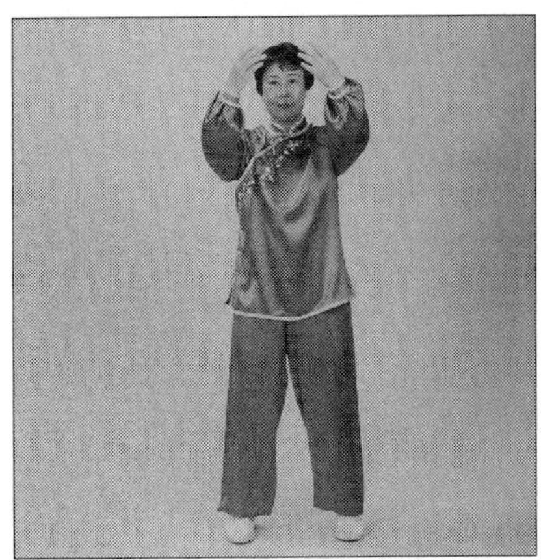

8 b. Arms continue to raise, as palms pass through the Upward Dantian.

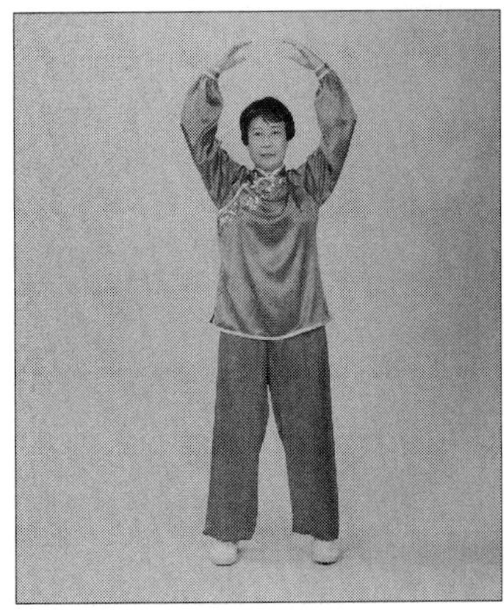

8 c-1. Arms continue to raise up above the head, until the Laogong point on the palms faces the Baihui point on the top of the head.

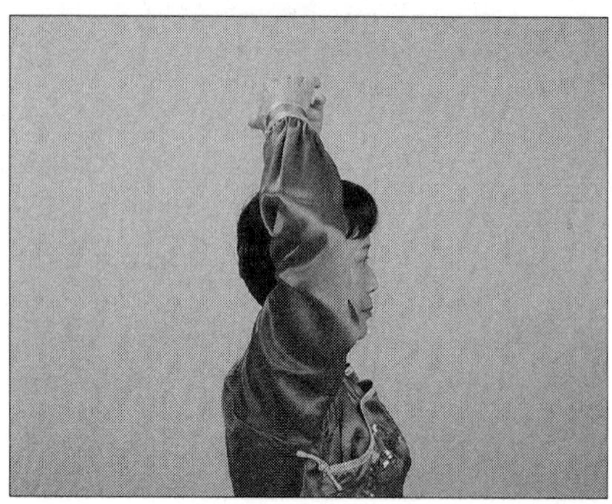

8 c-2. (ANOTHER ANGLE) This is the correct position to complete the form, Lift Arms. Notice the Laogong points on both palms face the Baihui point on the top of the head.

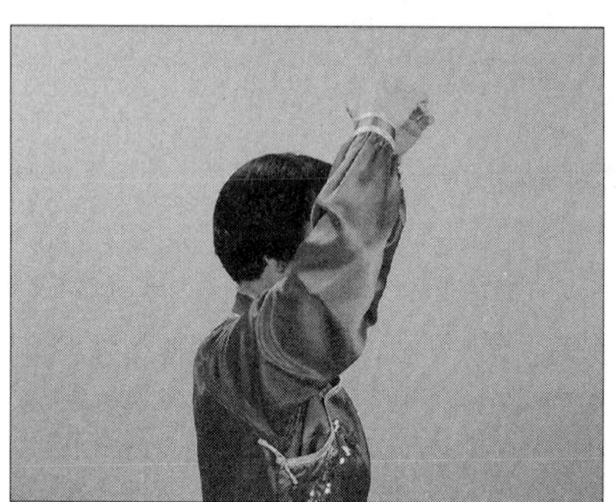

8 c-3. (ANOTHER ANGLE) This is an example of the arms and palms incorrectly placed to complete the form, Lift Arms. Here you can see the arms and palms are not gently brought back far enough to make the connection between the Laogong points on both palms and the Baihui point on the top of the head.

CHI ESSENTIALS: When the arms raise up, inside the arms is fresh Chi. With the Laogong point on both palms, guide fresh Yin energy to the Baihui point on the top of the head. Also while raising the arms upward, the Pericardium Channel is stimulated on the inside of the hands and arms, while the Triple Warmer Channel is stimulated on the outside of the arms and hands. While the hands raise up, both of the palms pass the Qihu point. There receive Chi, and allow the Chi to come to the Middle Dantian, down to the Lower Dantian, and continue down to the Yongquan point; as the hands go upward.

9. CLASP HANDS

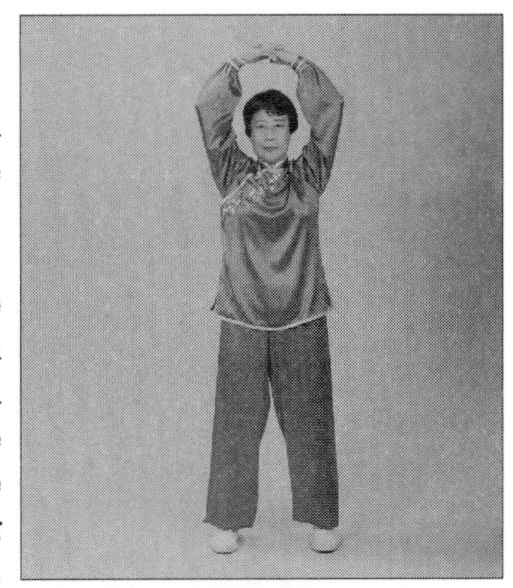

9. Interlace fingers, and clasp hands with palms (Both Laogong points) still facing the Baihui point on top of the head.

CHI ESSENTIALS: When interlacing the fingers, pour fresh Chi in the Baihui point on the top of the head. Bring the Chi to down through the Du and Ren meridians all the way to along the Kidney Channel to the Yongquan point. You may feel some pushing or downward pressure at the Baihui point. Also you may feel some warmth or tingling on the bottom of the feet and near the center of the ball of the foot at the Yongquan point. Both of these are perfectly natural, and are no cause for alarm.

10. TURN UP PALMS

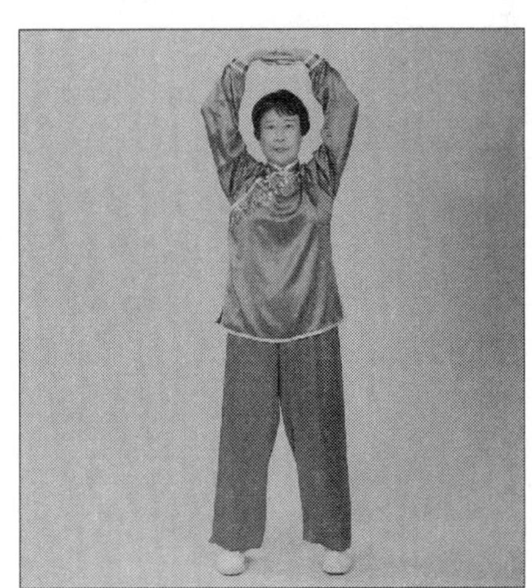

10 a. With hands still clasped, rotate elbows outward, and turn palms up toward the sky (Yang).

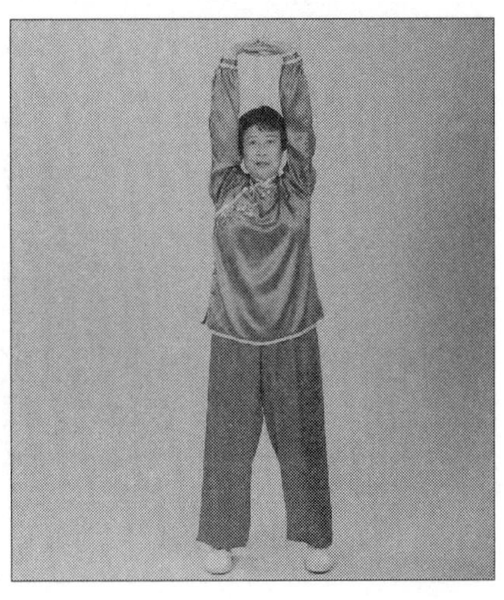

10 b. Then with the Yi (Mind), consciously press the palms firmly and gradually straight upward, while gradually straightening the arms and legs. Keep the feet planted firmly on the ground.

CHI ESSENTIALS: As the palms face up to the sky, you receive the Yang energy, while opening and stimulating the Du Meridian. As you stretch upward towards the sky, you continue to receive Yang energy, and the skeletal muscles, tendons, and connective tissue are stretched as well.

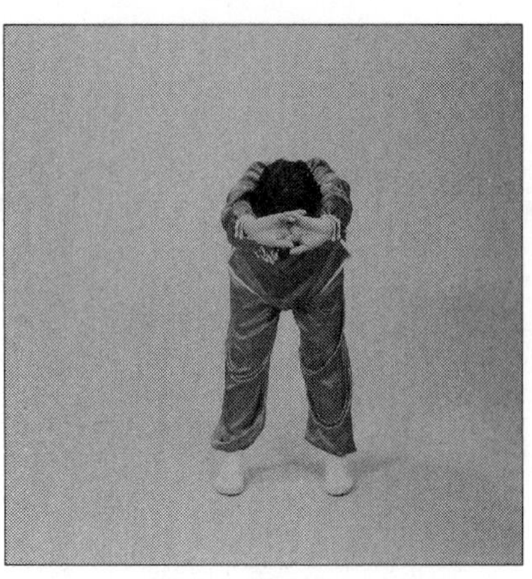

11. BEND WAIST (FORWARD, LEFT AND RIGHT)

11 a. With the hands still clasped, slowly bend the body forward at the waist, while keeping the legs straightened. CAUTION: Practitioners with high blood pressure or heart problems are advised to keep the head above the heart when bending over at all times. Do not allow the head to pass down below the heart.

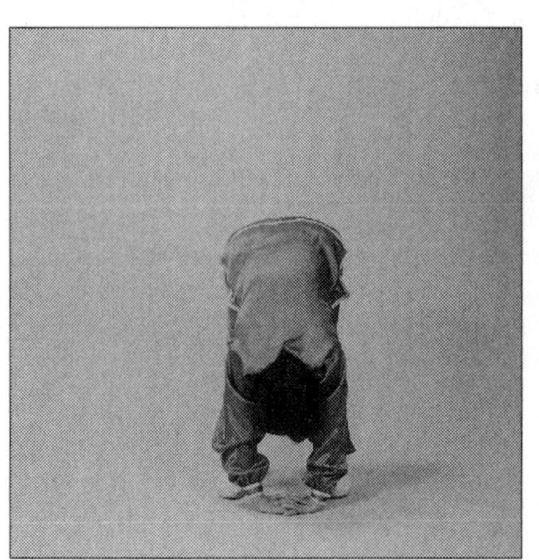

11 b-1. Press the palms on the ground gently between the two feet, or down as far as possible while keeping the legs straightened and knees locked. When bending down, keep the head in line with the torso. Also while bending over, do not bend the knees! If you cannot touch the ground, gently bend down a little more each day. In a relatively short time you will be able to touch the ground. Remember, it is not important whether you touch the ground or not. What's important is that the legs are straightened, the knees locked, and the palms stretch down as far as possible towards the ground; in order to stimulate the Bladder channel.

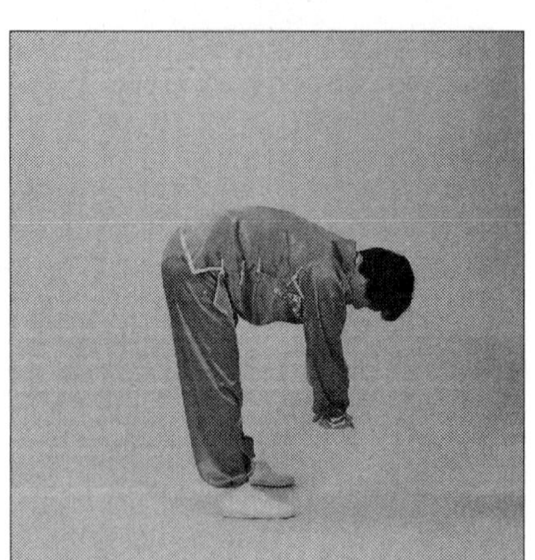

11 b-2. (ANOTHER ANGLE) Here is another correct example of Bend Waist without having to touch the ground. Notice the head stays in line with the torso allowing the chi to continue to flow to the head and throughout the body. Also notice that the legs remain straightened and the knees do not bend.

11 b-3. (ANOTHER ANGLE) Here's an incorrect example of bending the knees to touch the ground. By bending the legs to touch the ground, you have defeated the purpose for straightening the legs, which is to stimulate the Bladder Channel and strengthen the kidneys.

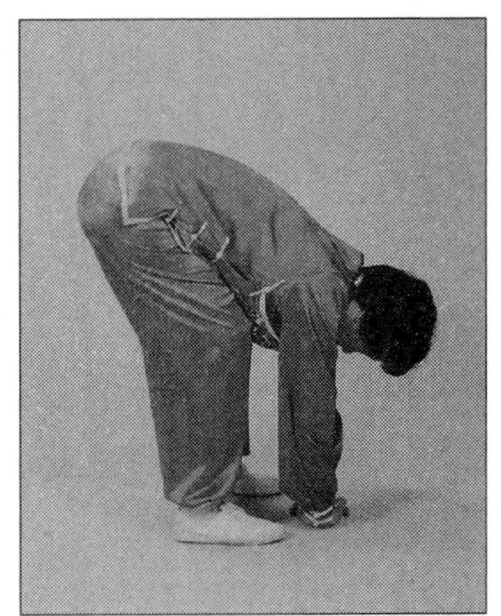

11 b-4. (ANOTHER ANGLE) Another incorrect example shows while the legs are straightened and the palms are nicely pressed on the ground, the neck is not aligned with the torso. Actually the neck is bent, causing the Chi to stop at the neck, and hindering the flow of Chi throughout the body.

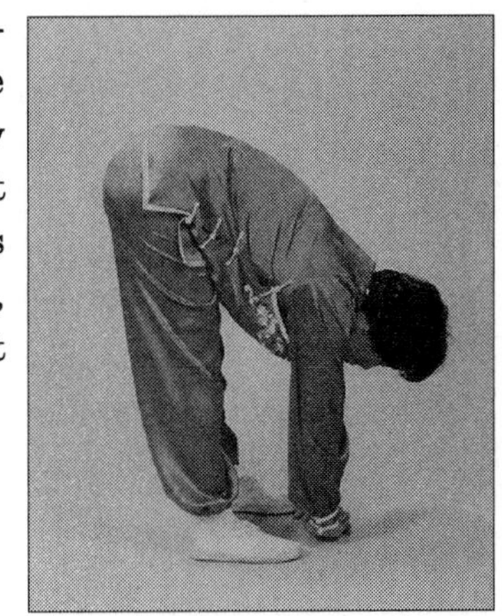

11 c. Then gently allow the torso to come up slightly from the ground, while maintaining straightened legs. However, when coming up relax the knees.

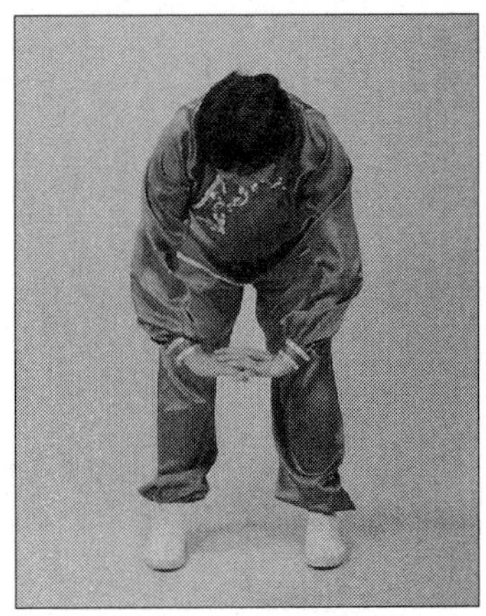

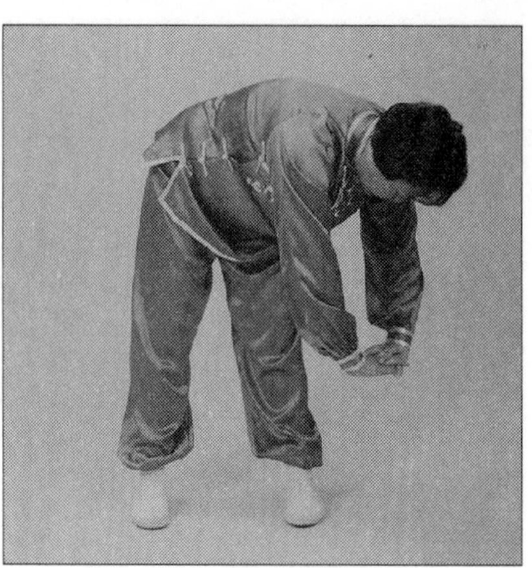

11 e. Then with the momentum of coming up slightly, turn your torso to the left.

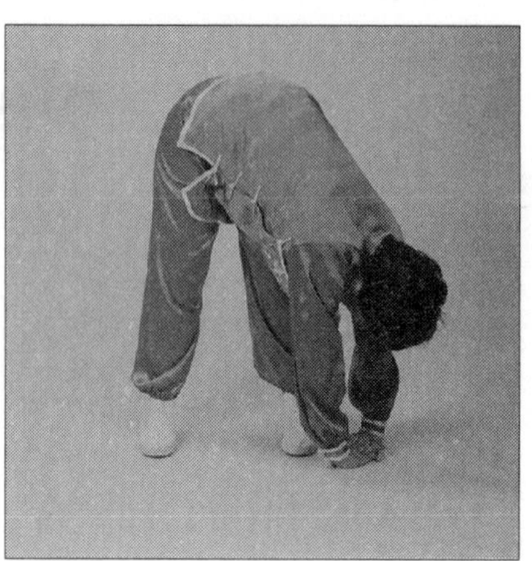

11 f. Press palms to the ground (or, as far down as possible), out in front of the left foot. Keeping your hands clasped, your legs straightened, and your knees locked. Do not bend the knees to touch the ground.

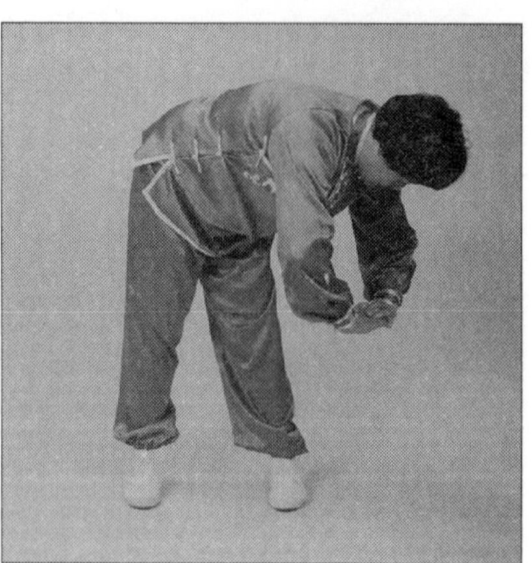

11 g. Then allow the torso to come up slightly, while maintaining straightened legs with relaxed knees.

11 h. With the momentum of the torso coming up, turn your torso to the right.

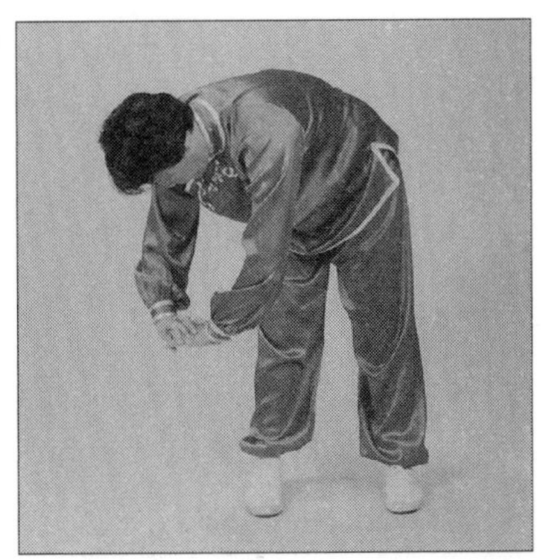

11 i. Then press palms to the ground (or, as far down as possible), out in front of your right foot. Keeping your hands clasped, your legs straightened, and your knees locked.

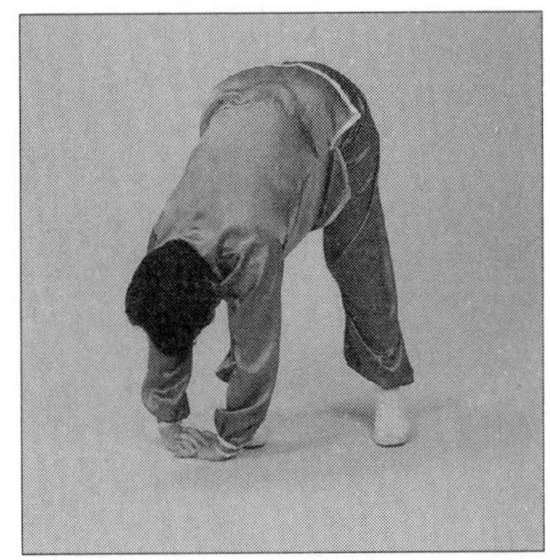

11 j. Then allow the torso to come up slightly, while maintaining straightened legs with relaxed knees.

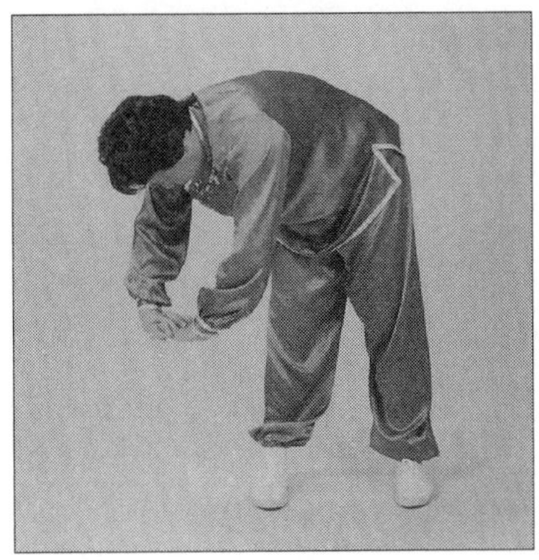

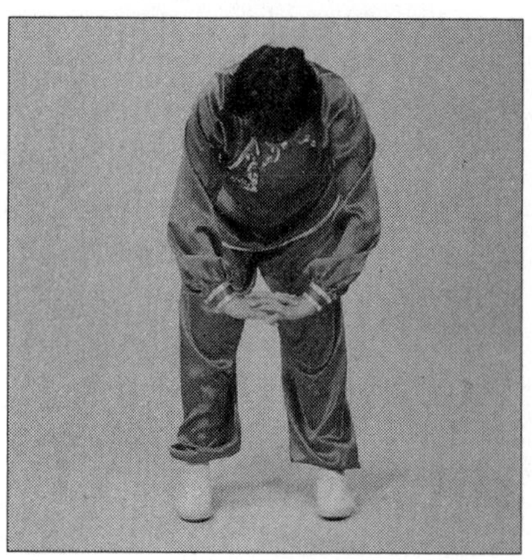

11 k. With the momentum of the torso coming up, bring your torso back to the center between your parallel stance.

CHI ESSENTIALS: As you bend at the waist forward, the Chi passes down to the Lower Dantian. As you bend further, you are bringing the Chi up the Du Meridian. When you relax each time after pressing down either towards or on the ground, you allow the Chi to flow down the Ren Meridian. Make sure you gently touch the tip of the tongue to the upper palate. By circulating the Chi on the Du and Ren Meridians together with the body's up and down movements, you are training the Pulmonary Circulation (Small Orbit). Also, receive the Earth's energy (Yin), as the two palms press down either towards or on the ground. CAUTION: If you have heart problems or high blood pressure, remember to not bend the head downward past the heart.

12. TWINE HANDS

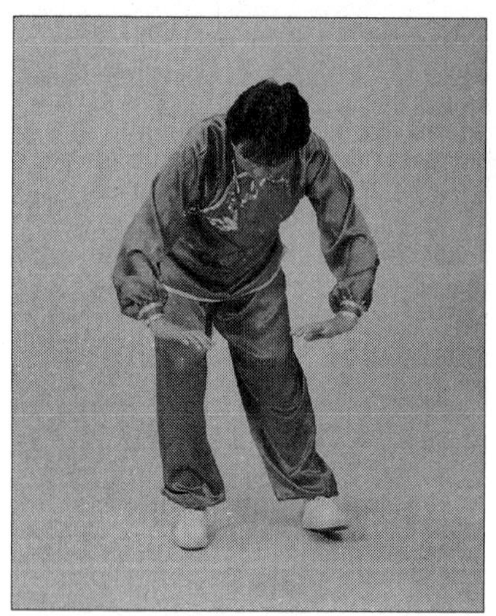

12 a. Separate the two hands with palms facing the earth and the fingers pointing towards each other. Eyes focus on the right hand. Simultaneously move the weight into the right foot, turn the waist left, and gradually begin turning the left toe to the left 90 degrees.

12 b. Continue pressing the palms outward freely to shoulder level, turning the waist gradually back to the right, while allowing the torso to come up. The left toe has completed turning 90 degrees to the left. The eyes follow the right hand. Don't twist the right knee.

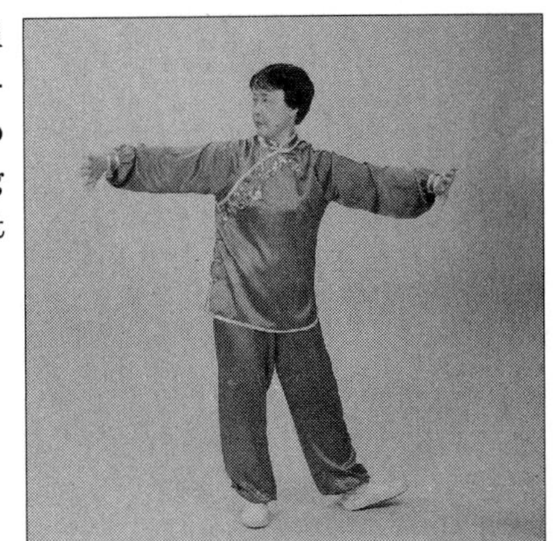

12 c. Then turn the waist back to the left gradually, while allowing the right arm to swing downward, left, and up to meet the outside of the left arm. As the right arm swings gradually turn the right arm inward, and gradually turn the left arm inward. The right forearm will vertically cross on the horizontal line of the outside of the left forearm. Make your movements smooth, and time the aforementioned movements to all begin and end at the same time.

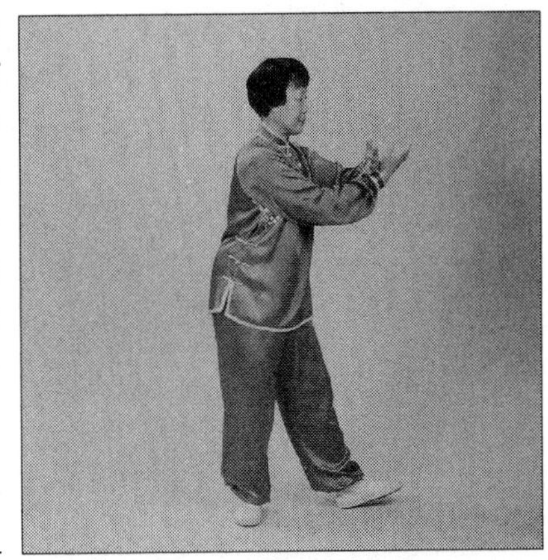

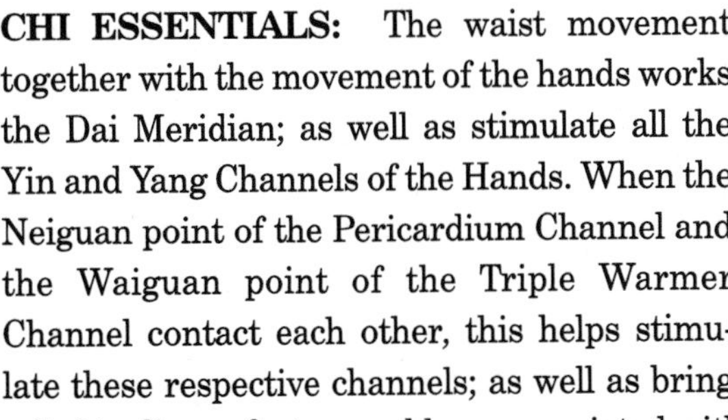

12 d. Then turn the waist, and hip slightly right, while bringing the right forearm over the left arm. Then turn the waist back to the left, to vertically cross the horizontal line of the inside of the left forearm.

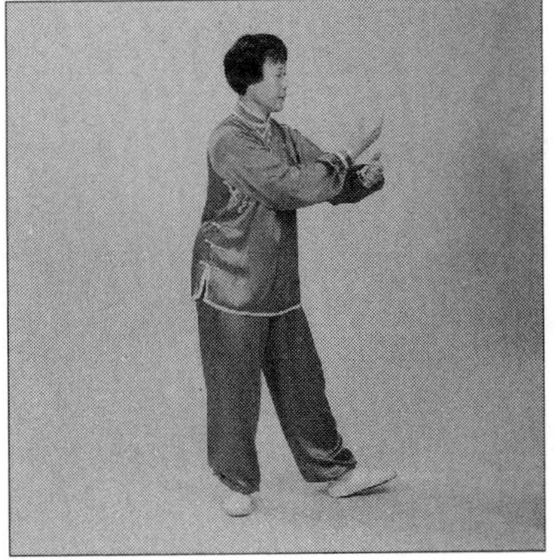

CHI ESSENTIALS: The waist movement together with the movement of the hands works the Dai Meridian; as well as stimulate all the Yin and Yang Channels of the Hands. When the Neiguan point of the Pericardium Channel and the Waiguan point of the Triple Warmer Channel contact each other, this helps stimulate these respective channels; as well as bring relief to discomfort or problems associated with the heart.

13. RECOVER AIR

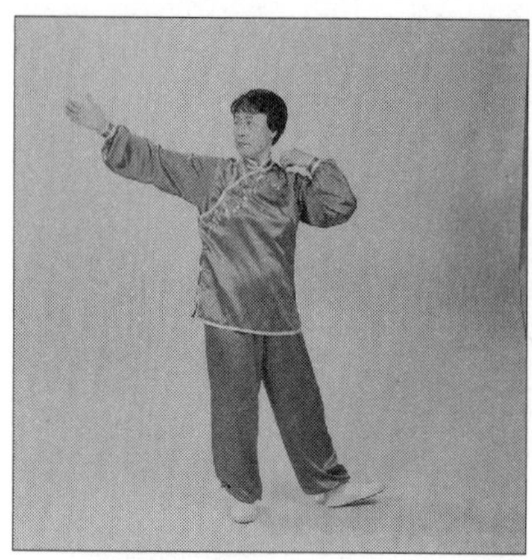

13 a-1. Bring the left arm down, back, and up, while turning the waist right. Simultaneously bring the fingers of the left hand together to form the Eagle's Beak, and place the drawn together fingers in the left Quepen point above the left collar bone.

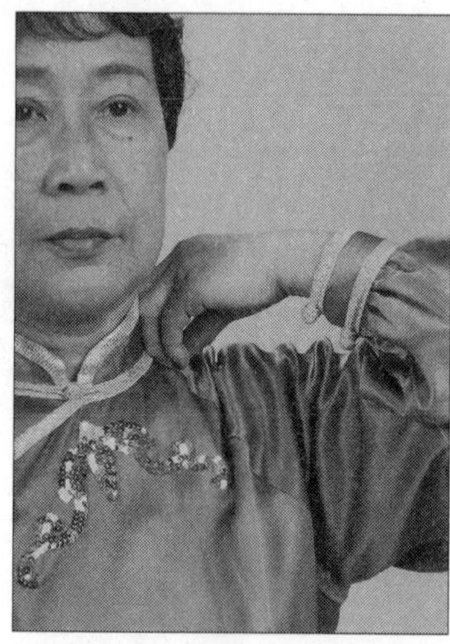

13 a-2. (ANOTHER ANGLE/CLOSE UP) As the Left Eagle's Beak contacts the Left Quepen, do not use force on this very sensitive point. Instead allow the drawn together fingers to rest on the Quepen point.

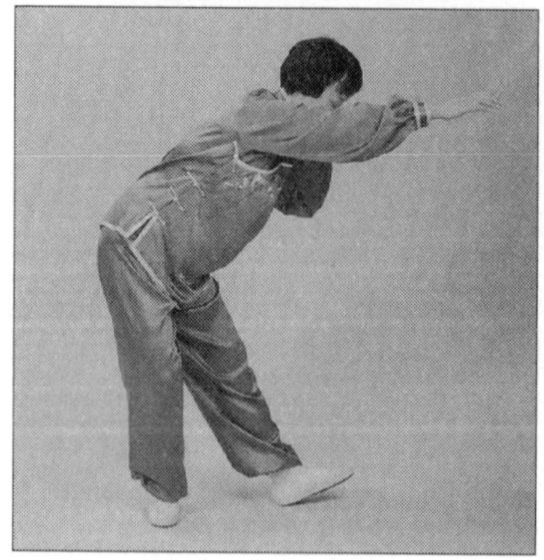

13 b. The right hand continues to travel up and over. Turn your waist gradually back to the left, while gradually bending at the waist down towards your left toes. As you bend over to grab the first two toes on the left foot, keep the right knee vertically aligned with the right toe.

CHI ESSENTIALS: With the Eagle's Beak, pour fresh Chi in the Quepen point. Allowing the Chi to pass through the Qihu, and come down to be stored in the Lower Dantian. As you bend at the waist over to grab the first two toes, the energy will naturally come up to the Huiying, Lower Dantian, and Middle

Dantian. Stimulating the Yin Channels of the Feet and Hands including the Liver, Heart, Spleen, Kidney, and Lung Channels.

14. PULL LEFT TOES (3 X)

14 a-1. Grip the first two toes of the left foot with the thumb, fore and middle fingers of the right hand. Keep the left Eagle's Beak in the left Quepen point. CAUTION: Remember to not bend the head past the heart if you have heart problems or high blood pressure. See 14 d-1 and 14 d-2 for an effective option in doing this posture.

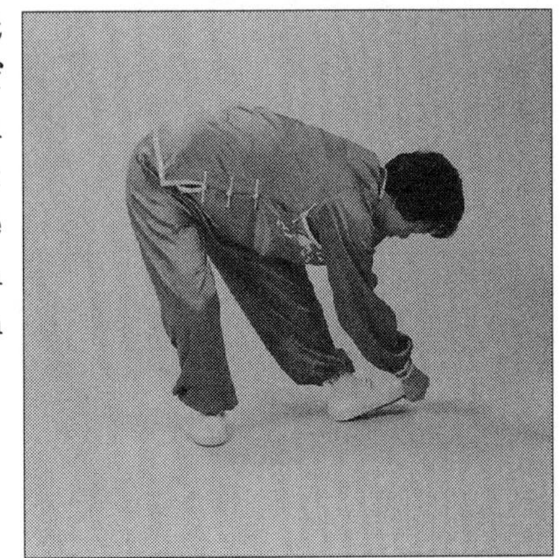

14 a-2. (ANOTHER ANGLE/CLOSE UP) The right thumb, pointing downward, grips the first two toes on the top side of the left foot . While the fore and middle fingers, pointing downward as well, grip the back-side of the toes. The ring and small finger gently curl into the palm to apply a more snug and specific grip on the first two toes.

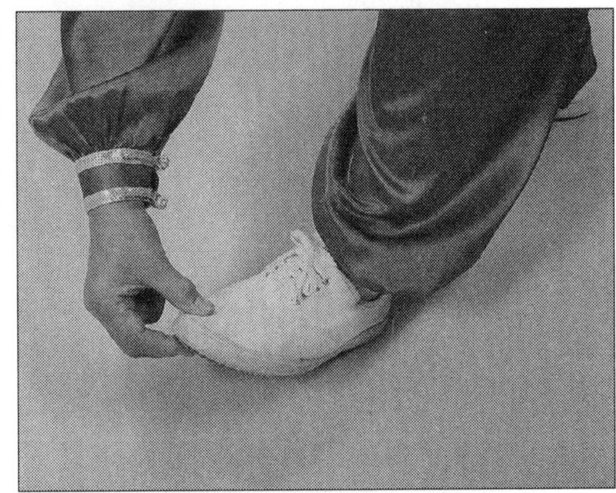

14 b. Gently pull the toes with the right hand, as the waist turns left. Keep the left Eagle's Beak in the left Quepen point. Keep both elbows relaxed. Allow the left elbow to turn back and up if possible while the right elbow bends each time the waist is turned to the left for a total of three times. Don't move the elbows without turning the waist. Furthermore, notice that the right knee maintains vertical alignment with the right toe at all times during this form.

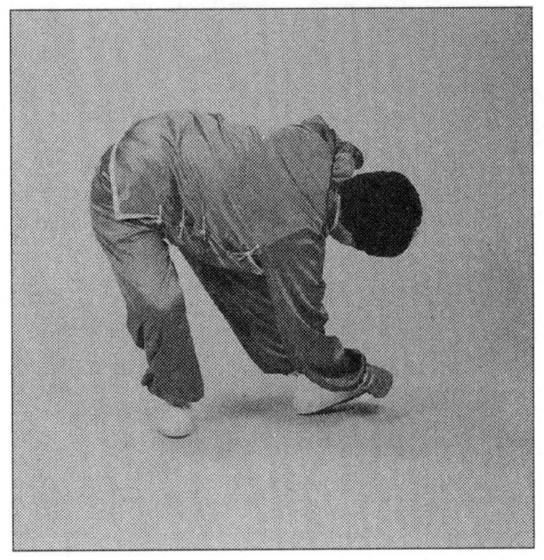

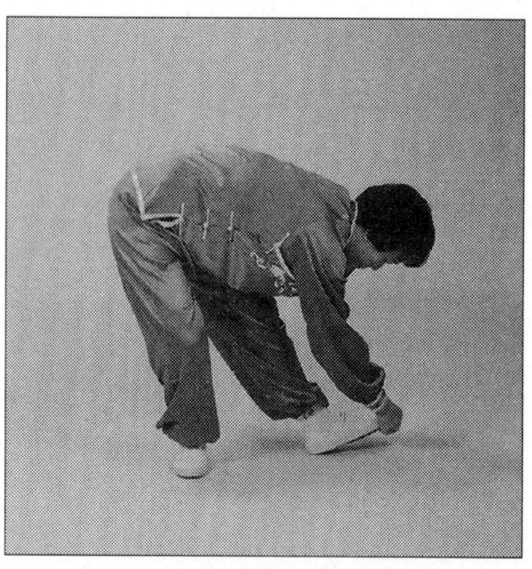

14 c. After turning the waist each time return to the position with your torso lined up with your left leg, and bent forward at the waist.

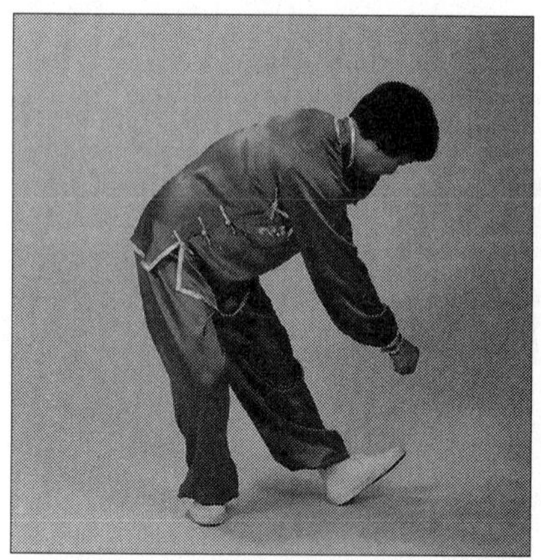

14 d-1. Here is an option of doing the form, Pull Left Toes (3x), correctly. If you are unable to grab the toes, bend downward and extend the arm as far down as you can. Notice the head stays in line with the torso, and the right knee is vertically aligned with the right toe. Use the Yi (Mind) to imagine your thumb, fore, and middle fingers grabbing the first two toes. Utilizing the Yi (Mind) to try to go down a little more each day. Don't try all at once to grab the toes if you are unable to do so.

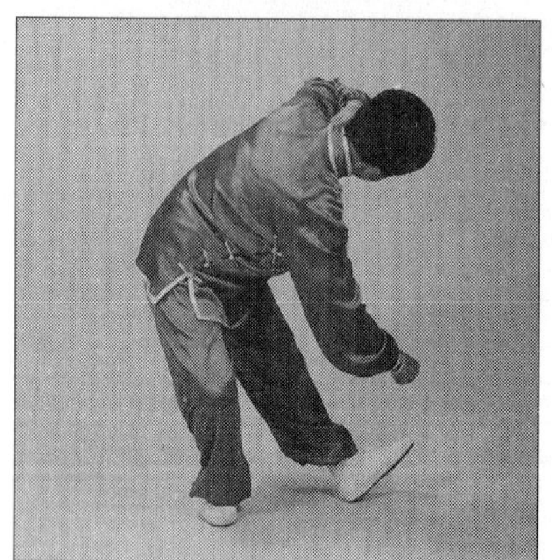

14 d-2. Notice as the waist turns in this option, that the left Eagle's Beak maintains contact with the Left Quepen point. The right hand maintains an imaginary grip on the left toes. Also notice that the right knee maintains vertical alignment with the right toe. Both elbows are relaxed. Allow the left elbow to come up and the right elbow to bend, when the waist turns. Don't move the elbows without turning the waist.

*Repeat movements 14 a-1 and 14 b (or, 14 d-1 and 14 d-2) two more times for a total of three times. Then do 14 c to contact the next form.

CHI ESSENTIALS: The action of twisting the waist stimulates the Stomach, Urinary Bladder, Gallbladder, Large, and Small

Intestine Channels; as well as working on the Yang channels to achieve balance together with the previous form.

15. PUSH AIR

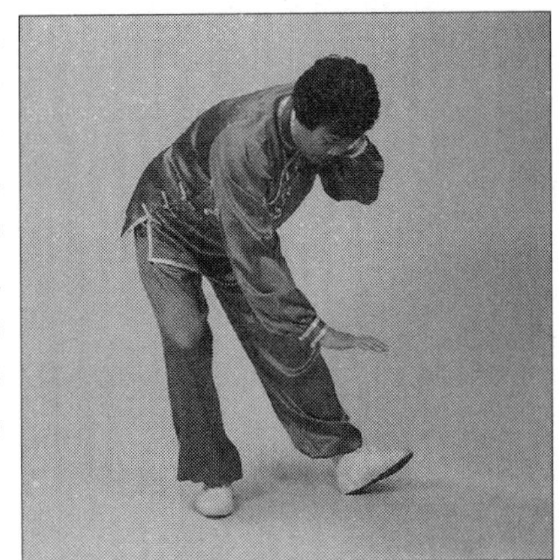

15 a. Let go of the left toes. Right hand forms a palm with the fingers slightly separated, while the left hand maintains the Eagle's Beak, and continues to contact with the left Quepen point. The eyes follow the right hand while the waist starts to turn right. Gradually push right palm to the right side, while simultaneously turning the left ball of the foot inward, parallel with the right foot.

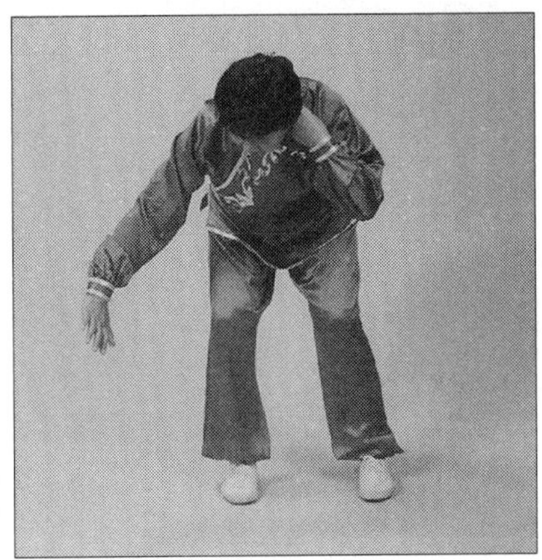

15 b. Continue watching and gradually pushing the right hand out to the side, until the left foot is parallel with the right, the Shenque point (Navel) faces slightly to the right of the center between the two feet, and the right elbow begins to lock up.

CHI ESSENTIALS: By pushing out the palm you are stimulating the Heart, Pericardium, Triple Warmer, and Small Intestine Channels, while simultaneously pulling out and dispelling bad Chi.

16. SCOOP UP AIR

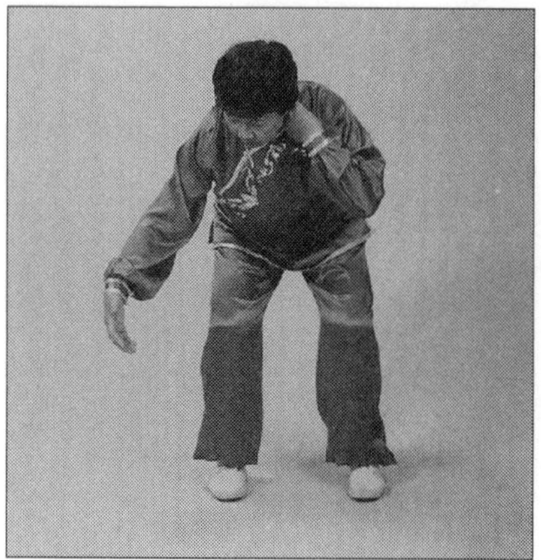

16 a. The left Eagle's Beak maintains contact with the left Quepen point. Continue pushing the right palm outward. Just as the right elbow starts to lock up, turn the right arm outward, relax the wrist, and turn the right fingers outward. After the palm circles outward, turn the right arm inward, and turn up the right palm up to form the Scooping palm.

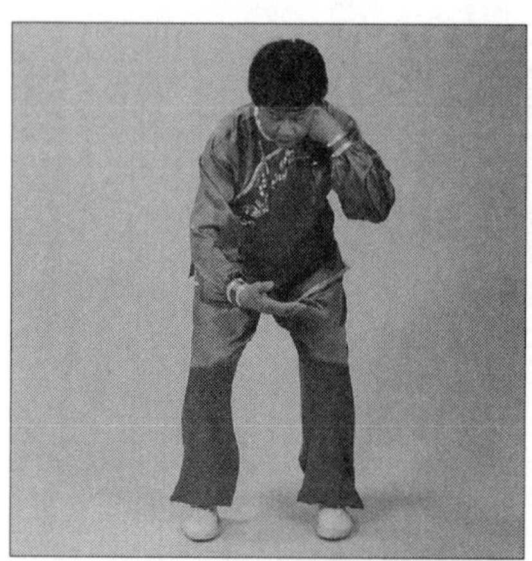

16 b. Continue watching the right Scooping palm, as you bring it slowly back to the center between the two feet. Gradually turn the waist slightly to where the Shenque point (navel) is facing slightly to the left of the center between the two feet. There finishing at the same time in one line just to the left of the center between the two feet are: the Shenque point (Navel), the right Scooping palm, and the eyes as they gaze at the right Scooping palm.

CHI ESSENTIALS: Receive fresh Qi with the Scooping palm, and pour it in the Quepen point with the Eagle's Beak. As you come up to stand erect, use the movement upward to bring the Chi down from the Quepen point, through the Qihu point, and store the Chi in the Lower Dantian.

17. TURN BODY AND RECOVER AIR

17 a. The left Eagle's Beak continues contact with the left Quepen point. Gradually bring the torso upright, allowing the right scooping palm to stay in the center, and follow the movement of the torso up. As the right hand comes up, gradually change the right palm into an Eagle's Beak. Place the right Eagle's Beak (where the four fingers grasp the thumb) in the right Quepen point.

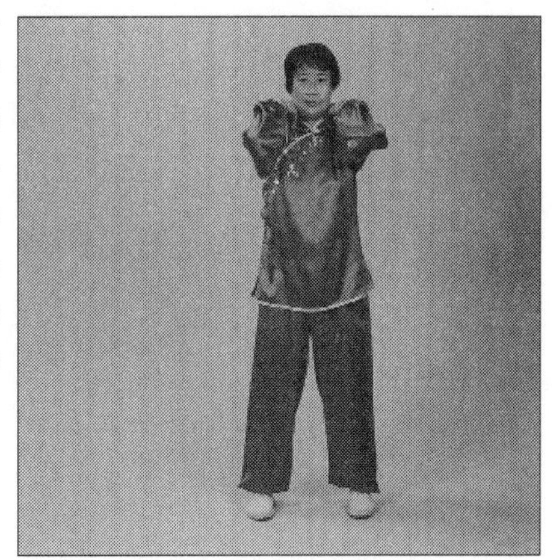

17 b. Then change the left hand from Eagle's Beak to palm, and extend the left hand outward, palm facing up. Simultaneously, turn the waist right, while raising the right toe, and turning the right foot 90 degrees outward to the right. Watch the left hand.

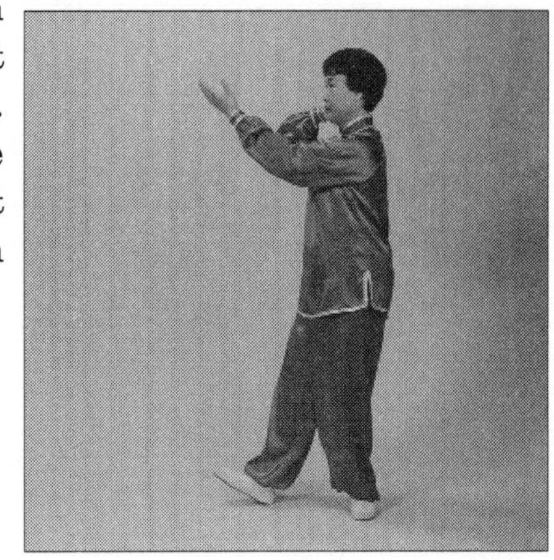

17 c. Then, gradually turn the waist back to the left, while letting the left arm swing down, back, and up. Continue watching the left hand.

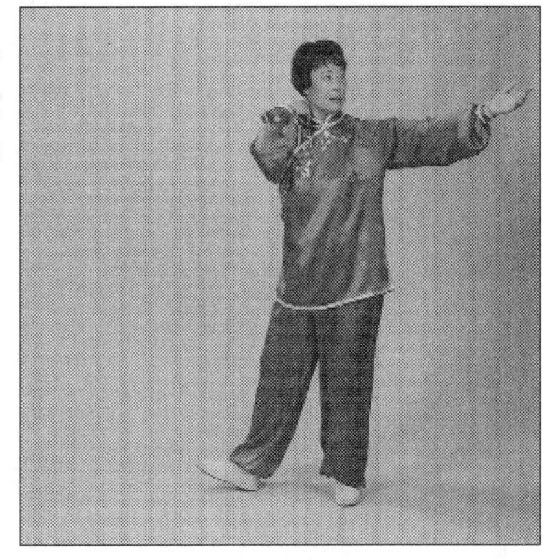

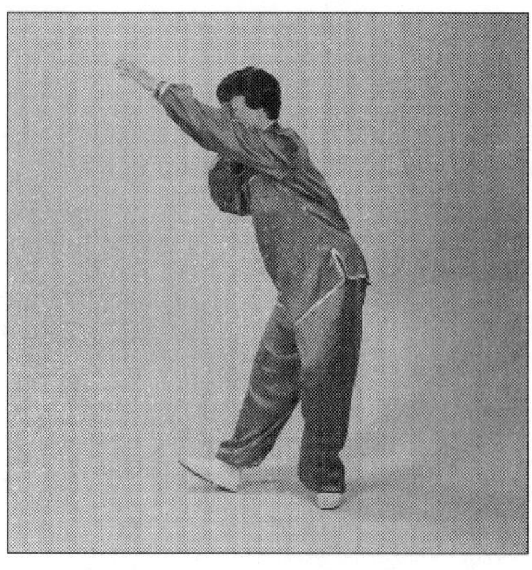

17 d. Continue to bring the arm over, while turning the waist back to the right. Bend at the waist over to grab the first two toes on the right foot with the left hand. Keep the left knee vertically aligned with the left toe.

CHI ESSENTIALS: See Chi Essentials for Form 13: RECOVER AIR.

18. PULL RIGHT TOES (3 X)

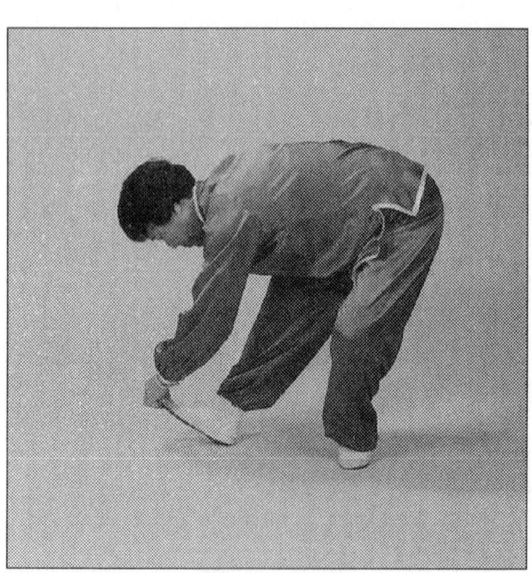

18 a. Grip the first two toes on the right foot with the thumb, fore, and middle fingers of the left hand. Keep the right Eagle's Beak in the right Quepen point. CAUTION: Do not bend the head past the heart if you have heart problems or high blood pressure. See 14 d-1 and 14 d-2 for an option for doing this posture. Change the directions for the left side to accommodate the right side.

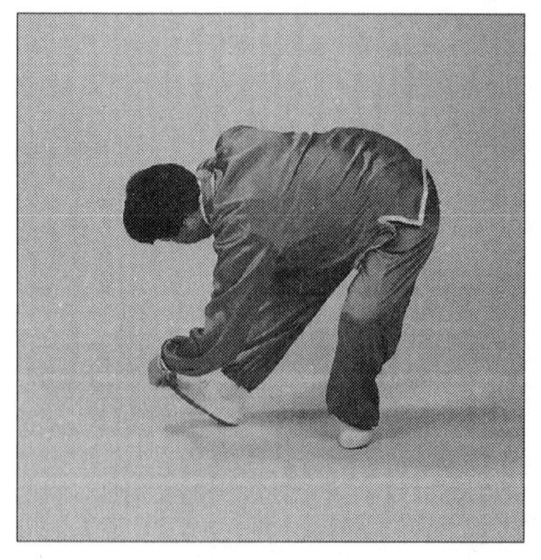

18 b. Opposite with the left side, gently pull the first two toes on the right foot with your left hand, as the waist turns right. Keep the right Eagle's Beak in the right Quepen point. Keep both elbows relaxed. Allow the right elbow to turn back and up, if possible, while the left elbow bends each time the waist is turned to the right for a total of three times. Don't move the elbows without turning the waist. Furthermore, notice that the left knee maintains vertical alignment with the left toe at all times during this form. Again, if you are unable to grip the first two toes on the right foot. See Forms 14 d-1 through 14 d-2 for a simplified yet correct version of Pull Toes, and perform the directions opposite with the right side. Remember don't force yourself to bend and grab your toes, until you are ready to do so. Gently bend a little more each day, and soon you will be able to do so. Remember here and throughout form's practice to not bend the head past the heart if you have heart problems or high blood pressure.

*Repeat movements 18 a and 18 b two more times for a total of three times. Then do 18 a again to contact the next move.

CHI ESSENTIALS: See Chi Essentials for Form 14: PULL LEFT TOES (3 X).

19. PUSH AIR

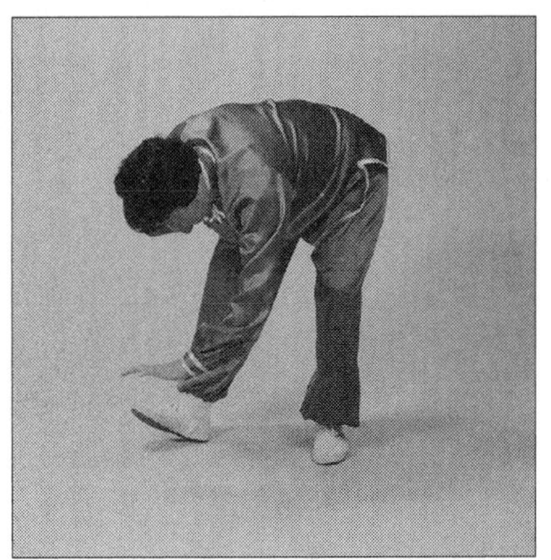

19 a. Opposite with Form 15, let go of the right toes. Left hand forms a palm with fingers slightly separated, while the right hand maintains the Eagle's Beak, and continues to contact with the left Quepen point. The eyes follow the left hand while the waist starts to turn left. Gradually push left palm to the left side, while simultaneously turning the right ball of the foot inward, parallel with the left foot.

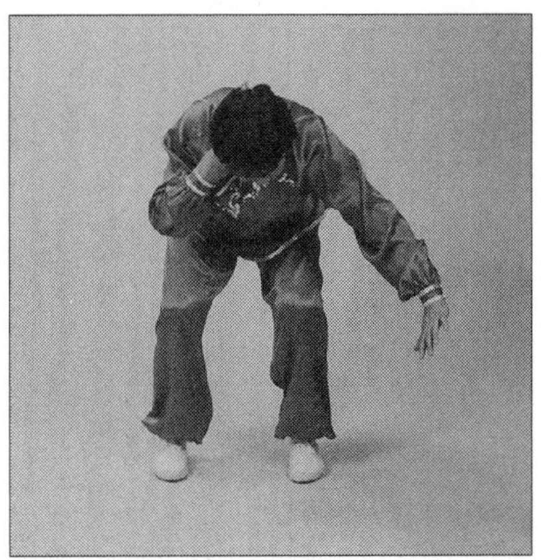

19 b. Continue watching and gradually pushing the left hand out to the side, until the right foot is parallel with the left, the Shenque point (navel) faces slightly to the left of the center between the two feet, and the left elbow begins to lock up.

CHI ESSENTIALS: See Chi Essentials for Form 15: PUSH AIR.

20. SCOOP UP AIR

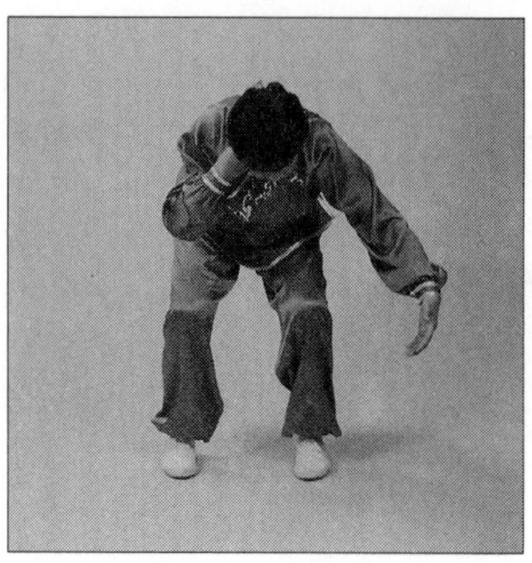

20 a. The right Eagle's Beak maintains contact with the right Quepen point. Continue pushing the left palm outward. Just as the elbow starts to lock up, turn the left arm outward, relax the wrist, and turn the left fingers turn outward. After the left palm circles outward, turn the left arm inward, and turn the left palm up to form the Scooping palm.

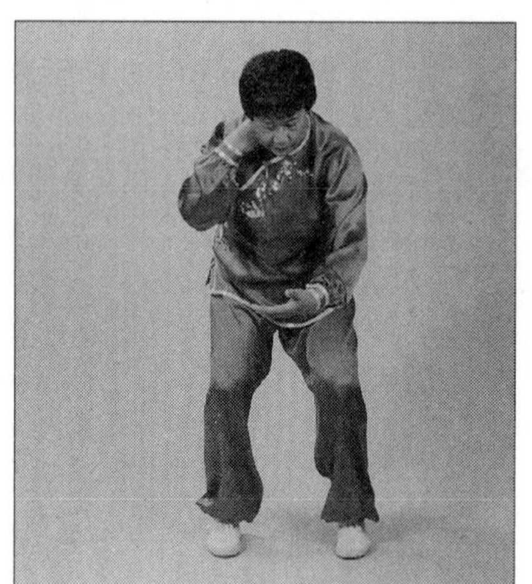

20 b. Continue watching the left Scooping palm, as you bring it slowly back to the center between the two feet. Gradually turn the waist slightly to where the Shenque point (Navel) is facing slightly to the right of the center between the two feet. There finishing at the same time in one line just to the right of the center between two feet are: the Shenque point (Navel), the left Scooping palm, and the eyes as they gaze at the left Scooping palm.

CHI ESSENTIALS: See Chi Essentials for Form 16: SCOOP UP AIR.

21. TWINE HANDS

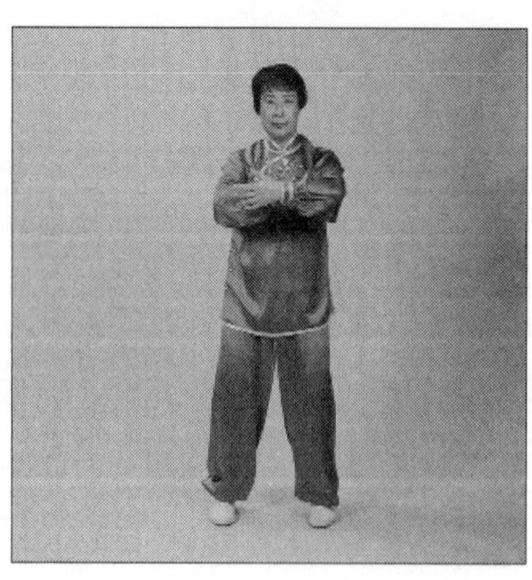

21 a-1. Gradually bring the torso upright, while gradually changing the right Eagle's Beak to the palm, bring the right palm down to where the right Laogong point faces inward to the left nipple, and the fingers on the right hand point left. Simultaneously, the left hand comes, faces inward with the Laogong point on the left hand facing the right nipple. Use the shoulder blades to extend forward slightly to round the arms.

21 a-2. (CLOSE UP) The left forearm is in front of the right forearm, and both arms are horizontal. The arms are slightly rounded, and if properly aligned the right Waiguan point will be facing the left Neiguan point.

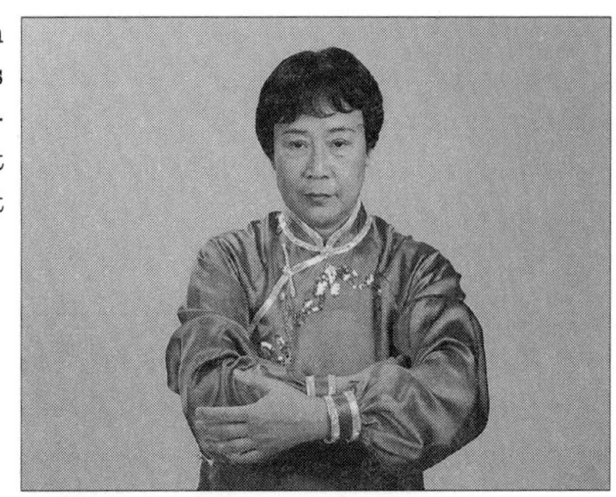

21 b. (The following movements 21 b through 21 e are continuous and evenly paced) Then turn the waist gradually left, while gradually bringing the right forearm under the left forearm and the left forearm above the right forearm.

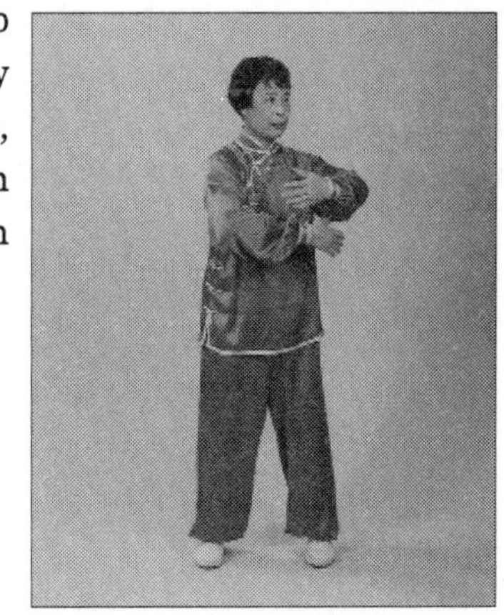

21 c-1. Then turn the waist gradually back right to the starting position, while gradually bringing the right forearm up to and in front of the left forearm and the left forearm down and behind the right forearm.

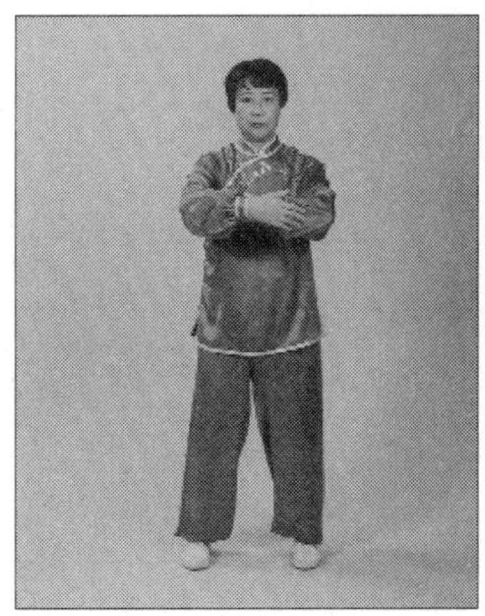

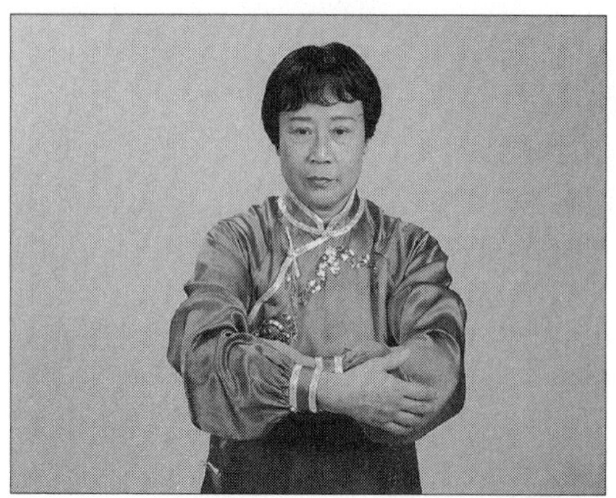

21 c-2. (CLOSE UP) The right forearm is in front of the left forearm, and both arms are horizontal. The arms are slightly rounded, and if properly aligned the left Waiguan point will be facing the right Neiguan point.

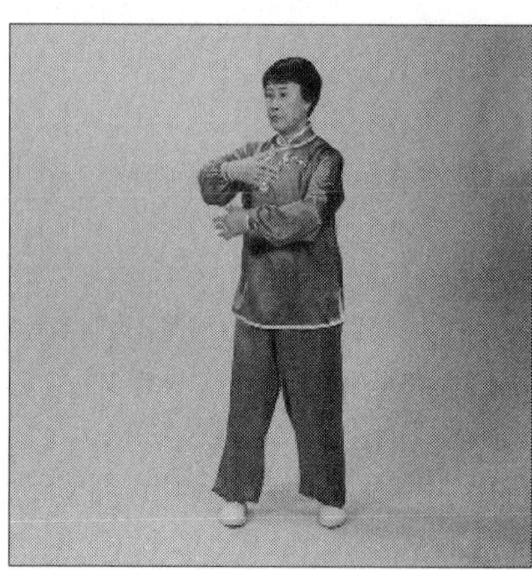

21 d. Then turn the waist gradually right, while gradually bringing the left forearm under the right forearm and the right forearm above the left forearm.

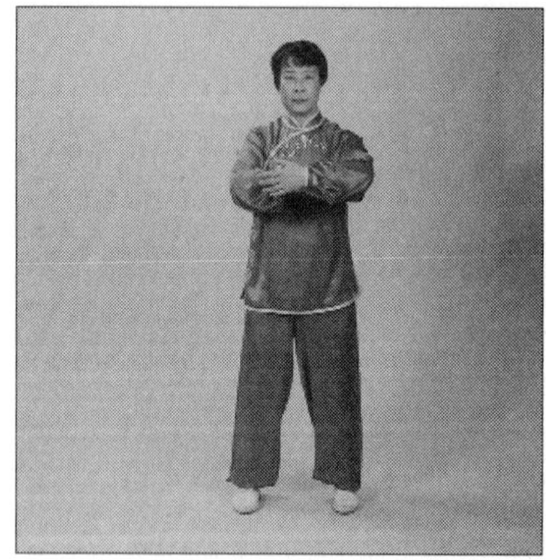

21 e. Then turn the waist gradually back left to the starting position, while gradually bringing the left forearm up to the front of the right forearm and the forearm down and behind the left forearm. Lining up the right Waiguan point with the left Neiguan point.

CHI ESSENTIALS: Turning the waist stimulates the Dai meridian which stimulates the Chi on all channels. The Neiguan point of the Pericardium Channel and the Waiguan point of the Triple Warmer channel circulate and contact each other, stimulating these two respective channels, and relieving any discomfort or problems associated with the heart. The movement of the arms turning inward toward the chest encourages the storage of Chi in the Middle Dantian.

22. WAVE HANDS LIKE CLOUDS (RIGHT, LEFT, AND RIGHT)

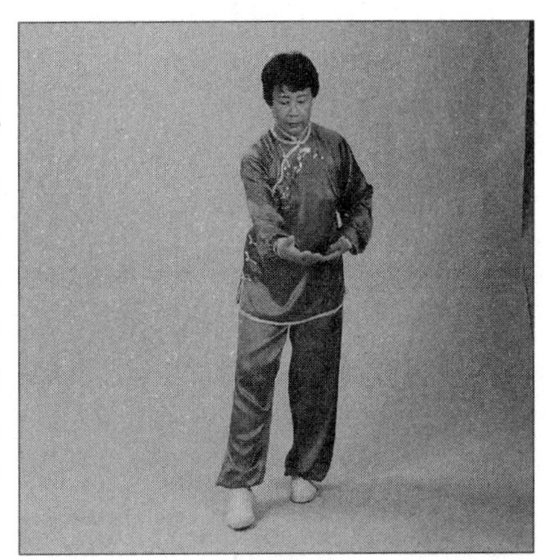

22 a. WAVE RIGHT HAND Turn waist left, while bringing the right hand under the left hand. Bring the left hand down to in front of the left Tianshu point. The left palm faces upward and slightly inward towards the left Tianshu point. The right foot extends forward, assuming a Right Empty Stance (Outer Edge of the Foot) with the outer edge of the right foot resting on the ground. Simultaneously, extend the right hand forward, palm up, to the left side, and watch the right palm.

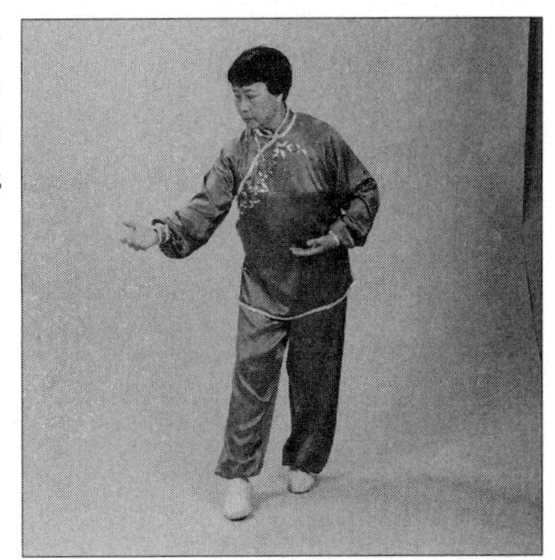

22 b. Turn the waist right, horizontally circle the hand to the right on a curve. Eyes continue watching the right palm, until the palm comes back 135 degrees to the right from the front.

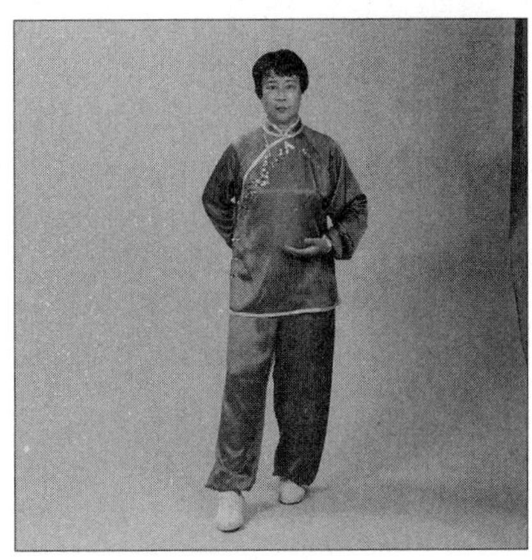

22 c-1. Then, gradually turn the waist left (back to the front), while simultaneously bringing the Hegu point on the right hand to contact the right Shenshu point. The left hand is still obliquely facing the left Tianshu point, while the right Empty stance (Outer Edge of the Foot) is maintained. The eyes look forward.

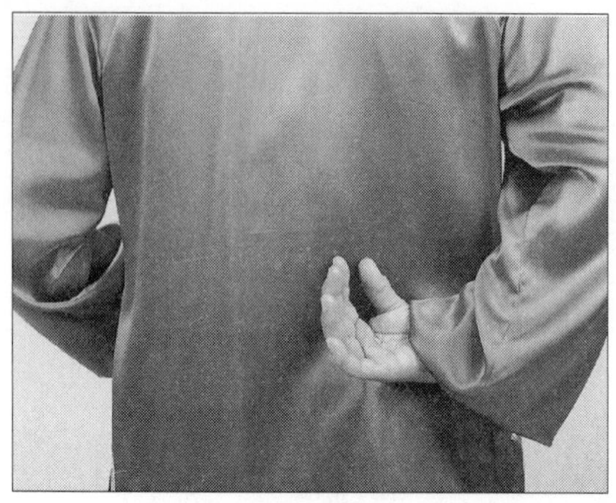

22 c-2.(REVERSE ANGLE/CLOSE UP) The fingers of the right hand point upward while the edge of the right forefinger rests on the superficial aspect of the Urinary Bladder Channel; in order that the right Hegu point can contact the right Shenshu point.

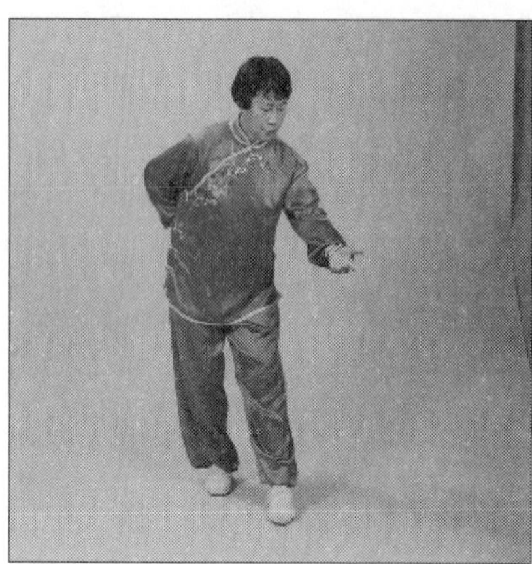

22 d. WAVE LEFT HAND Turn the waist right, and move the weight forward into the right foot. Extend the left hand forward and to the left, palm up, from the left Tianshu point. Simultaneously, extend the left foot forward lightly into the left Empty Stance (Outer Edge of the Foot). Turn the waist to the left, while horizontally circling the hand to the left on a curve. Eyes watch the left palm, until the palm comes back 135 degrees to the left from the front. Then the eyes look forward.

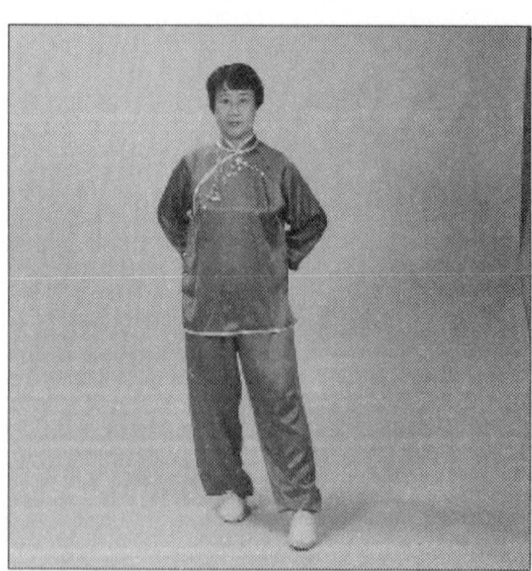

22 e-1. Then, gradually turn the waist right (back to the front), while simultaneously bringing the Hegu point on the left hand to contact the left Shenshu point. The right Hegu point on the right hand still contacts the right Shenshu point, while the left Empty stance (Outer Edge of the Foot) is maintained.

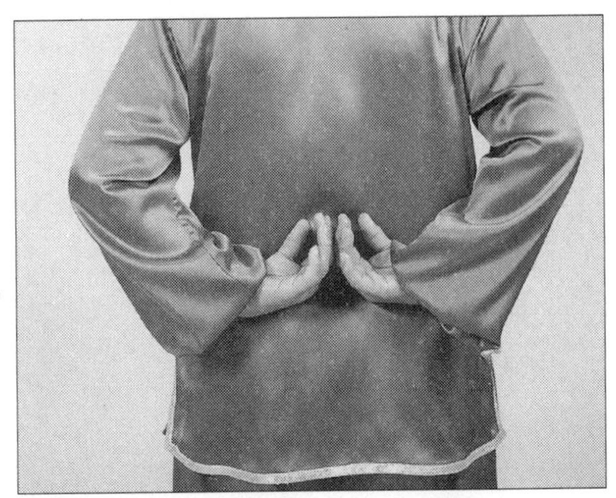

22 e-2. (REVERSE ANGLE/CLOSE UP) The fingers on both hands point upward, while the edge of both forefingers rest on the superficial aspect of the Urinary Bladder Channel; in order that the Hegu points on both hands can contact the Shenshu points on both sides of the body. Notice the right Hegu point contacts the right Shenshu point.

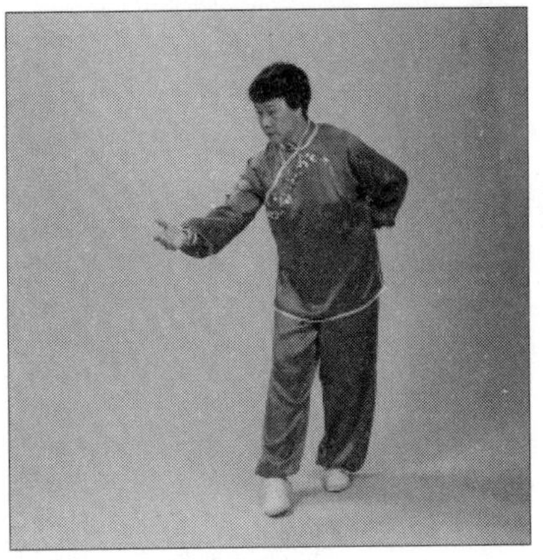

22 f. WAVE RIGHT HAND Turn the waist left, and move the weight forward into the left foot. Extend the right hand forward and to the right, palm up, from the right Shenshu point. Simultaneously, extend the right foot forward lightly into the right Empty Stance (Outer Edge of the Foot). Turn the waist to the right, while horizontally circling the hand to the right on a curve. Eyes watch the right palm, until the palm comes back 135 degrees to the right from the front. Then, turn the waist gradually left (back to the front), while bringing the Hegu point on the right hand to contact the right Shenshu point. Again both of the Hegu points on both hands contact both of the Shenshu points on both sides of the body (See Reverse Angle/Close Up: Form 22 e-2 for more visual and descriptive information.). Maintain the right Empty stance (Outer Edge of the Foot), while the eyes look forward.

CHI ESSENTIALS: First, the Laogong point on the left hand contacts the left Tianshu point stimulating the Stomach channel. The turning of the waist works the Dai Meridian, stimulating both the Yin and Yang channels of the body. When the eyes follow the palm, the Laogong point is activated and Chi is gathered. Simultaneously, when the outer edge of the foot contacts the ground, the Yongquan point located near the center of the ball of the foot is activated, and Yin energy is contacted and absorbed. The placing of the Hegu in the Shenshu point stimulates and helps store Chi in the Kidney, as well as the Urinary Bladder Channel. The entire form itself coordinates the waist movement with movements of the upper and lower limbs, thereby stimulating all Yin and Yang Channels on the feet and hands.

23. TWIST WAIST

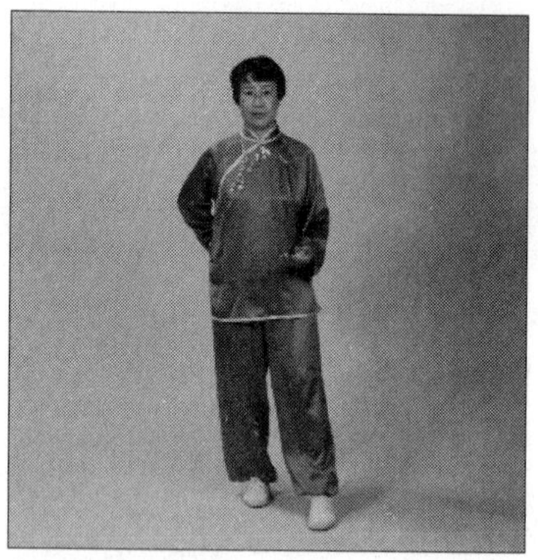

23 a. Turn the waist slightly right, and move the wait forward gradually into the right foot. Extend left foot forward lightly. Assuming the Empty stance (Ball of the Foot), while extending the left hand forward, palm up, with the left elbow staying close to the left side of the waist. Eyes look forward. The Hegu point on the right hand still maintains contact on the right Shenshu point.

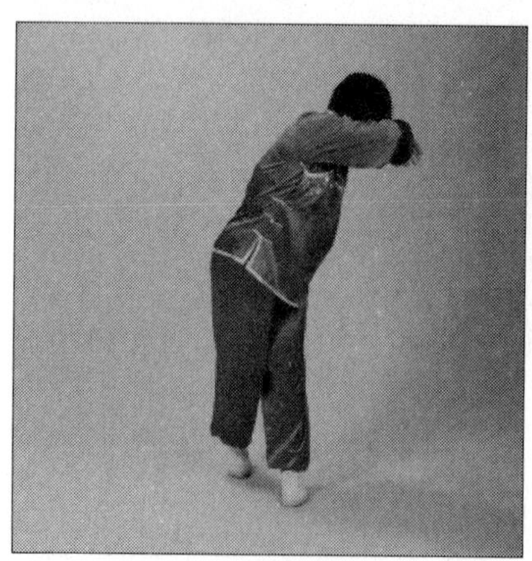

23 b-1. Twist the waist gradually left, while gradually raising both heels off the ground. The left hand circles horizontally to the left to the Huantiao point on the left hip. The right hand circles horizontally from the right Shenshu point to the Yintang point located between the eyebrows. Do not contact the superficial aspect of the points mentioned here. Keep a distance that is comfortable, and you can sense the magnetic connection of the points.

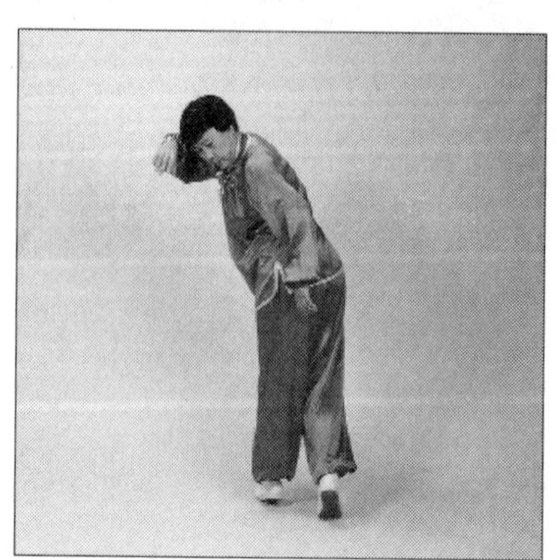

23 b-2. (REVERSE ANGLE) Notice both heels are off the ground, the fingers on both hands point downward. Twist the waist and look back at the back of the left heel.

23 b-3. (ANOTHER ANGLE/CLOSE UP) The Hegu point on the right hand faces the Yintang point located between the eyebrows.

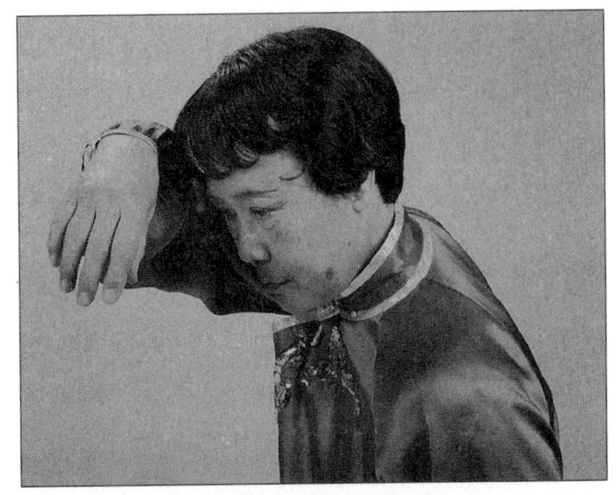

23 b-4. (ANOTHER ANGLE/CLOSE UP) The Hegu point on the left hand faces the Huantiao point on the left hip.

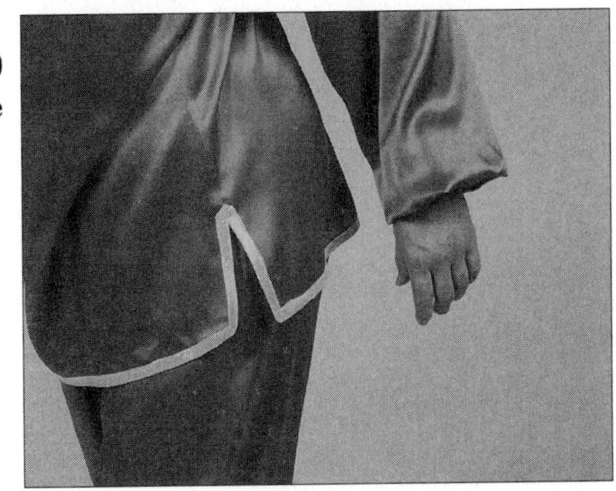

23 b-5. (ANOTHER ANGLE/CLOSE UP) Both heels raise off the floor gradually as high as possible. Because momentum carries the weight forward as you twist, the left or back heel will probably be able to raise higher. Prepare for the HEELS ON THE GROUND (FORCE METHOD).

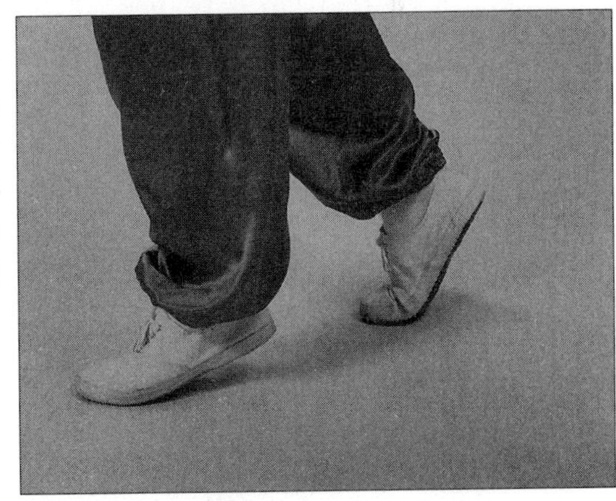

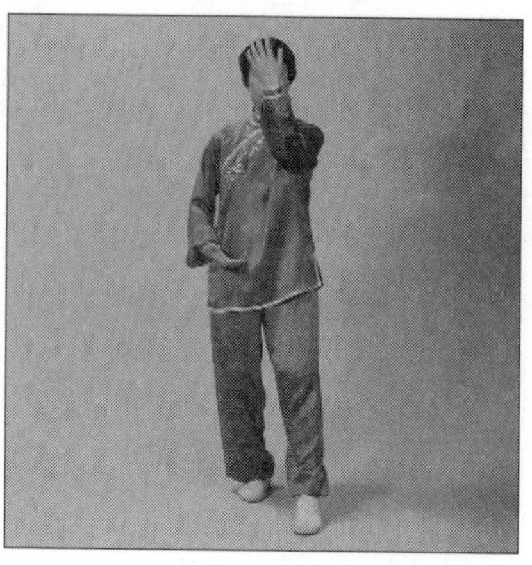

23 c-1. Then suddenly drop the right heel down with the force of all the body's weight. Simultaneously, the Laogong point on the left hand faces the Yintang point located between the eyebrows, while the right hand obliquely faces the right Tianshu point. The left foot is extended forward, and the left Empty stance (Ball of the Foot) is assumed.

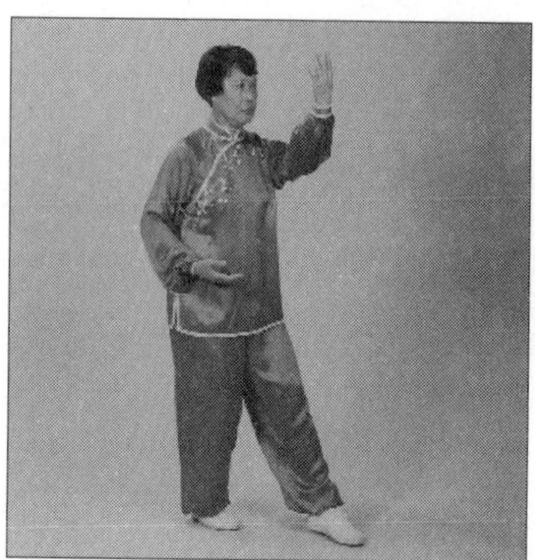

23 c-2. (ANOTHER ANGLE) The Laogong point on the left hand faces the Yintang point without holding any tightness in the left shoulder. The right hand faces the right Tianshu point without holding any tightness in the right shoulder. The elbow on the right hand rests on the right side of the waist.

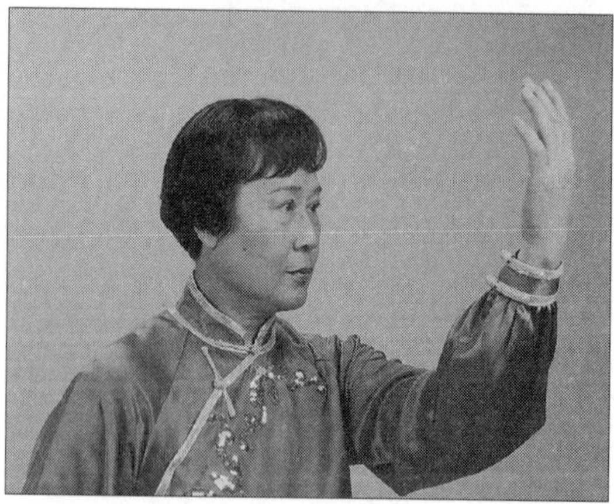

23 c-3. (ANOTHER ANGLE/CLOSE UP) Looking at the Laogong point in the left palm helps activate the Chi for emission from the Laogong point.

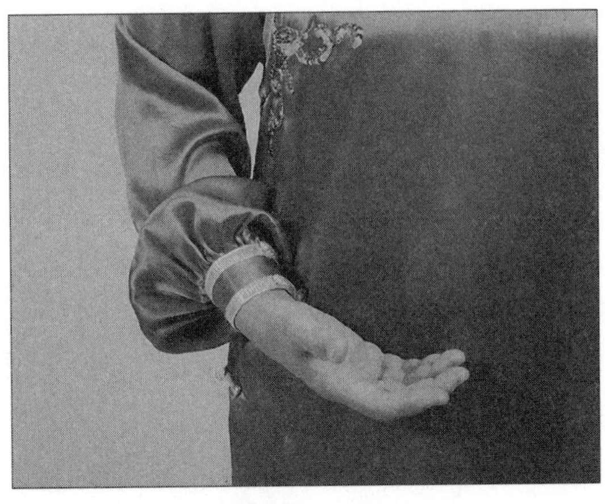

23 c-4. (ANOTHER ANGLE/CLOSE UP) The right palm obliquely faces the right Tianshu point.

CHI ESSENTIALS: Twisting the waist works the Dai Meridian which works both the Yin and Yang Channels of the body. The purpose of lining up the Hegu points with the Yintang and Huantiao points serves two purposes. First fresh Chi is stored in the Yintang and Huantiao points. Second, when the right heel comes down with the Heels Down (Force) method, a sudden shock is created that helps bring the Yang energy up and the Yin energy down to more effectively dredge the channels and bring out the bad chi.

The Laogong point on the left hand faces the Upward Dantian at the Yintang point. Looking at the Laogong point helps to collect fresh Chi at the Laogong point, that is then poured into the Upward Dantian.

24. DROP ARM TO RECOVER AIR

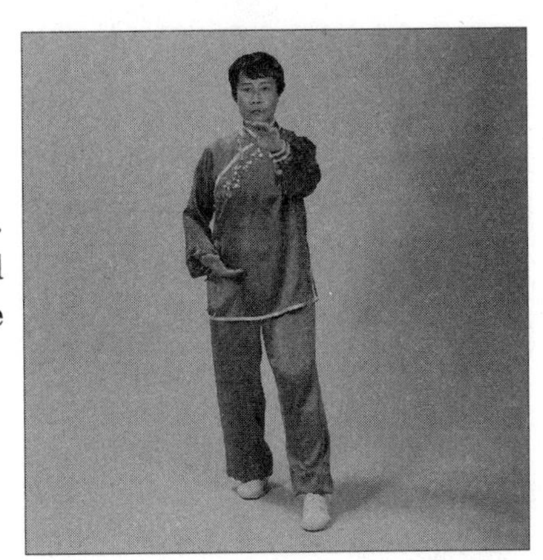

24 a. Gradually rotate the palm outward. Then gradually move the weight forward into the left leg, while gradually bringing the palm down.

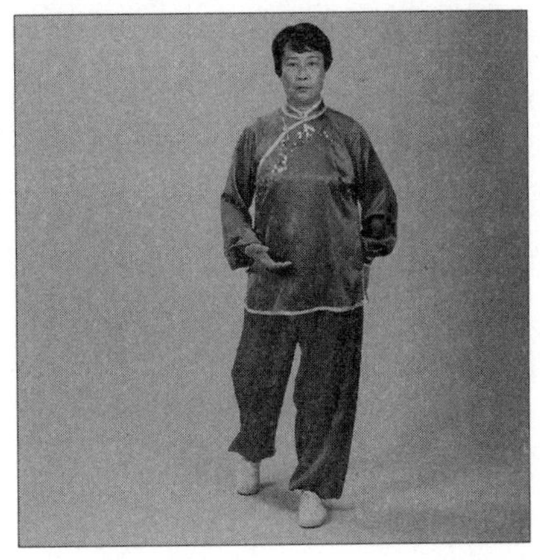

24 b-1. By the time the weight finishes coming forward and the back right heel raised off the ground, the palm should complete coming all the way down and the Hegu point on the left hand placed on the Huantiao point located on the left side buttocks.

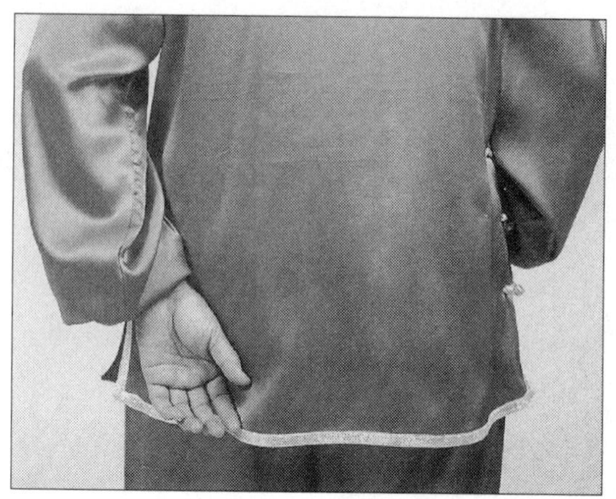

24 b-2. (REVERSE ANGLE/CLOSE UP) Notice the fingers on the left hand point downward. Making the contact of the Hegu point on the left hand to the Huantiao point located on the left side of the buttocks comfortable and natural.

CHI ESSENTIALS: When the left hand comes all the way down, the fresh Chi poured into the Upward Dantian at the Yintang point in the previous form, the Chi is brought down to the Lower Dantian. When the weight moves forward onto the left foot, and the back right heel raised, this encourages the Chi to come down to the Yongquan point as well. The Hegu point on the left hand packs fresh Chi on the Gallbladder Channel when contacting the Huantiao point located on the left side of the buttocks.

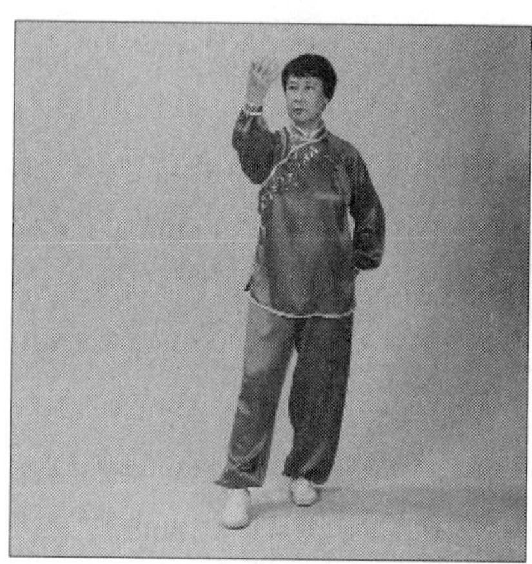

25. SPREAD SINGLE WING

25 a. Gently extend the right foot forward forming the Empty Stance (Ball of the Foot), while raising the right palm. The Laogong point on the right hand faces the Upward Dantian at the Yintang point between the eyebrows. Don't allow the shoulders to come up when raising the right hand, or when slightly turning the waist right. Look at the right palm.

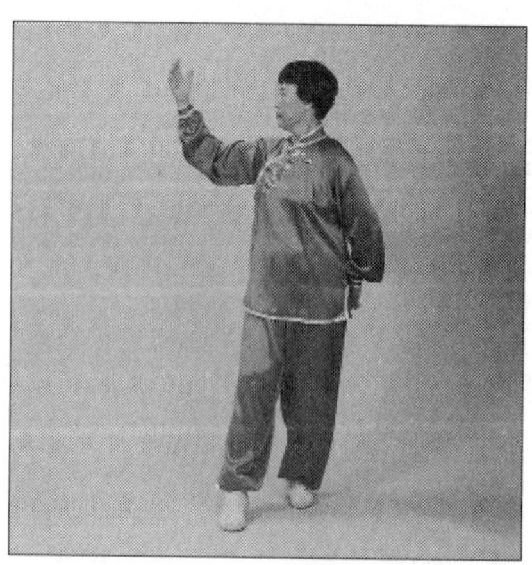

25 b. Gradually turn the waist right, while maintaining eye contact with the right palm. Maintain the vertical angle on the right arm, as the right arm turns horizontally back 135 degrees from the front. The Hegu point on the left hand maintains contact with the Huantiao point on the left side of the buttocks.

25 c-1. Gradually turn the waist left (back to the front), while bringing the Hegu point on the right hand to contact the right Shenshu point. Look forward and maintain your balance.

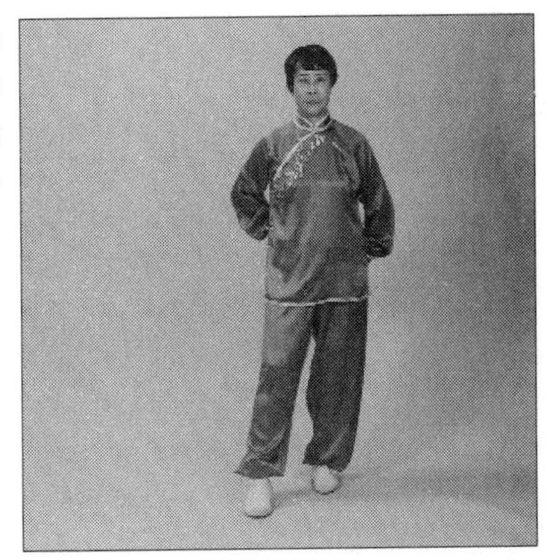

25 c-2. (REVERSE ANGLE/CLOSE UP) The fingers on the right hand point upward while the edge of the right fore finger rests on the superficial aspect of the Urinary Bladder Channel; in order that the right Hegu point can contact the right Shenshu point. The fingers on the left hand point downward making it easier and more natural for the Hegu point on the left hand to contact the Huantiao point located on the left side of the buttocks.

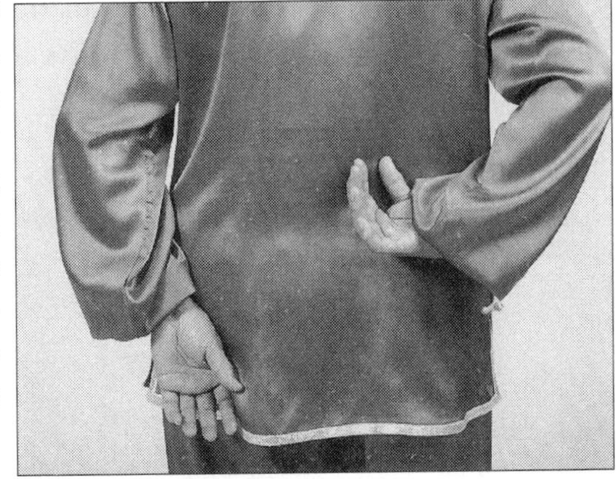

CHI ESSENTIALS: Pour fresh Chi into the Yintang point/Upward Dantian when the Laogong point on the right hand comes up to face the Yintang point located between the eyebrows. As the waist turns right, allow the Chi to pass through the right Qihu point located just below the collar bone in line with the right nipple, and continue all the way down to be stored in the Lower Dantian. The waist turning works the Dai meridian, which stimulates both the Yin and Yang channels of the body.

When the Hegu point on the right hand contacts the right Shenshu point fresh Chi is poured in and the Urinary Bladder Channel stimulated. The Hegu point on the left hand rests at the Huantiao point located on the left side of the buttocks continuing to stimulate the Gall Bladder Channel.

26. STEP FORWARD AND EXTEND ARM

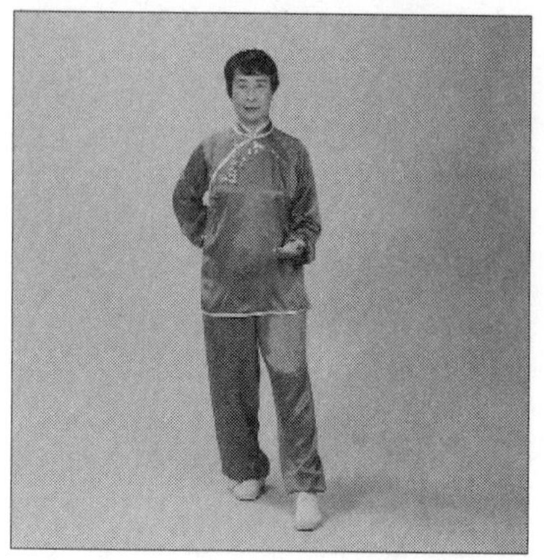

26. Gradually move the weight forward into the right foot. With forward momentum, gently extend the left foot forward forming the left Empty Stance (Ball of the Foot), while extending the left arm, palm up, with the left elbow contacting the left side of the waist.

The Hegu point on the right hand maintains contact on the right Shenshu point. Look forward and maintain your balance.

CHI ESSENTIALS: The Hegu point on the right hand maintains contact on the right Shenshu point to continue stimulating and warming the Urinary Bladder Channel. Allow the stimulation to continue all the way down to the ending point on the Urinary Bladder Channel at the Yongquan point located near the center of the ball of the foot. The left hand extends forward, and faces upward to collect fresh Chi. The ball of the left foot extends forward in the left Empty Stance (Ball of the Foot) and contacts the Earth's Energy (Yin).

27. WIND HAND AROUND HEAD AND EARS

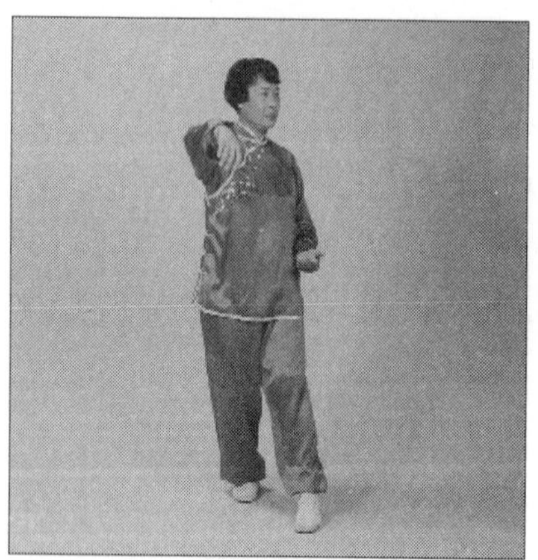

27 a. Gradually turn the waist left, while bringing the right hand from the right Shenshu point to the left. The fingers point downward, while the eyes look out connected with the waist's turning to the left. The left palm continues facing upward, while the left elbow maintains contact with the left side of the waist.

27 b-1. The right hand continues to the left, until the right hand meets the left ear. The eyes look back left 135 degrees from the front. The left Empty stance is maintained (Ball of the Foot).

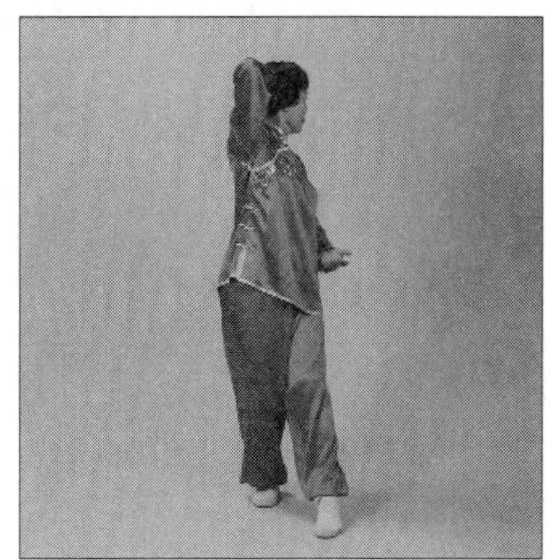

27 b-2. (REVERSE ANGLE/CLOSE UP) The fingers on the right hand point left, and contact the Triple Warmer Channel (Ermen point) in front of the ear.

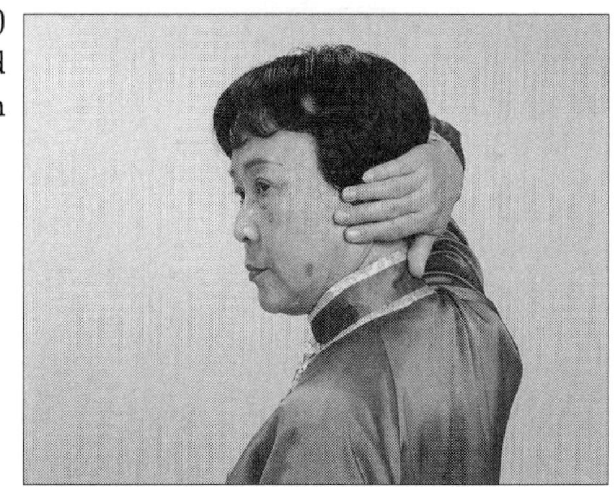

27 c-1. Gradually turn the waist right (back to the front), while allowing the right hand to come to the nape of the neck. Maintain the left Empty stance (Ball of the Foot), and the eyes follow the waist movement. Look forward, and maintain balance.

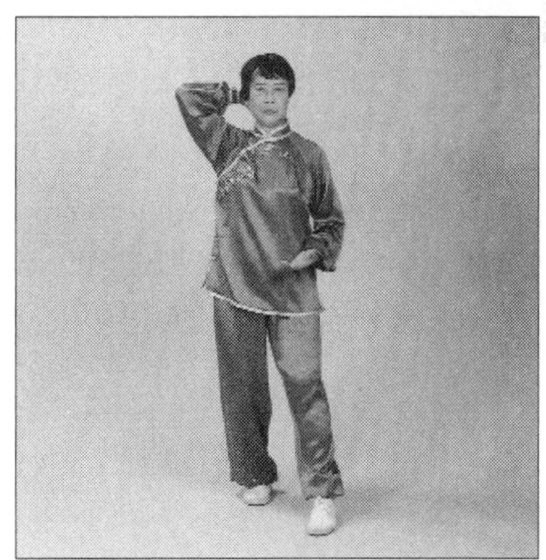

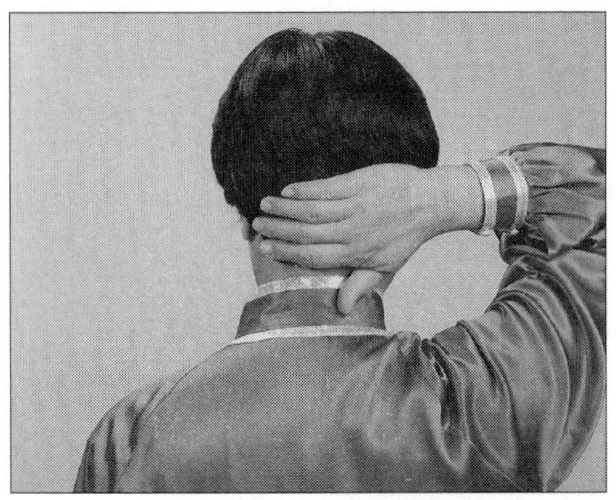

27 c-2. (REVERSE ANGLE/CLOSE UP) The fingers on the right hand still point left, and contact the Yangwei Meridian (Fengchi point).

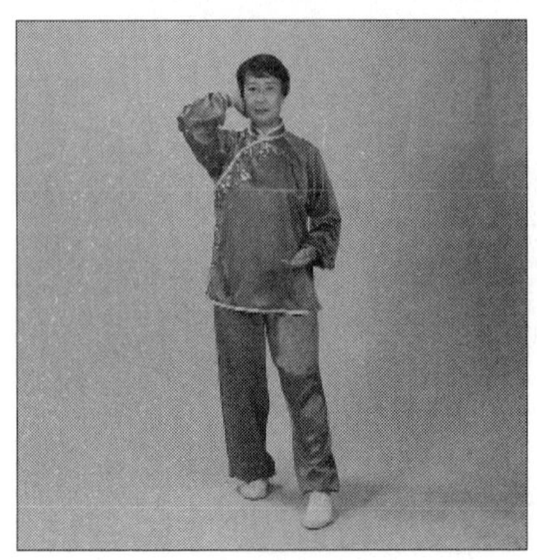

27 d. Finally, allowing the right shoulder to come down, which brings the right palm to the right ear. The elbow points to the front right. Look straight ahead.

CHI ESSENTIALS: The waist turning works the Dai meridian, which stimulates both the Yin and Yang Channels of the body. Bringing the fingers on the right hand to the front of the left ear stimulates the Ermen point, as well as the Triple Warmer Channel. The unwinding of the waist helps move the hand without isolated force. The fingers on the right hand contact and stimulate the Yangwei Meridian at the left Fengchi, Yamen, and Fengfu points (Points located all around the back edge of the hairline). Relaxing the right shoulder, helps naturally bring the right hand over to continue contacting and stimulating the Yangwei Meridian (Right Fengchi point). The palm on the left hand obliquely faces the left Tianshu point. Continuing to stimulate and warm the Channels on the left leg; especially the Stomach Channel. Allow the Chi to come all the way down to the toes. Especially to the big toe at the Yinbai point, thereby connecting with the Spleen Channel.

28. PRESS DOWNWARD

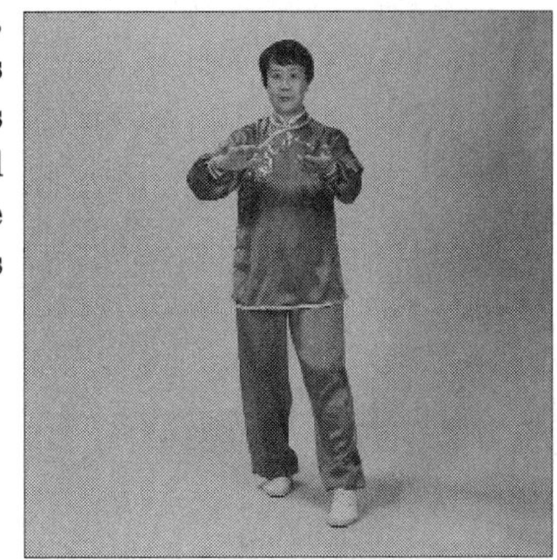

28 a. Gradually bring the right palm down, and the left palm up to where the palms pass level with the Middle Dantian. The fingers point slightly inward creating slightly flexed fingers and wrists. The left Empty stance (Ball of the Foot) is maintained. The eyes look forward.

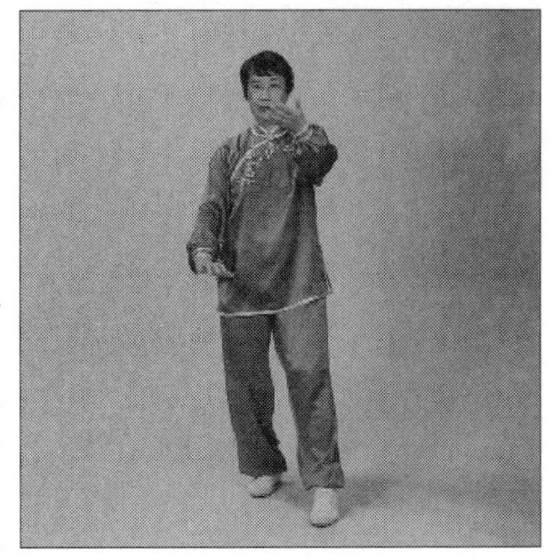

28 b. Continue bringing the left hand up to shoulder level, and the right hand down to hip level. Continue utilizing the left Empty stance (Ball of the Foot). The eyes look forward.

CHI ESSENTIALS: When the hands first move and pass, they are encouraging the bad chi to be expelled that may have been brought to the surface from the last movement of Wind Hand Around Head and Ears. Simultaneously, this movement stimulates the Kidney and Gallbladder Channels. Then after the hands pass each other, fresh Chi is gathered. The right hand also guides Chi to go down to the Lower Dantian for storage purposes, while the left hand comes up gathering fresh Yang Chi. The left heel remains up in the left Empty stance (Ball of the Foot), stimulating the Yongquan point. Encouraging the left side of the body to receive the Earth's energy (Yin).

29. PROP UP

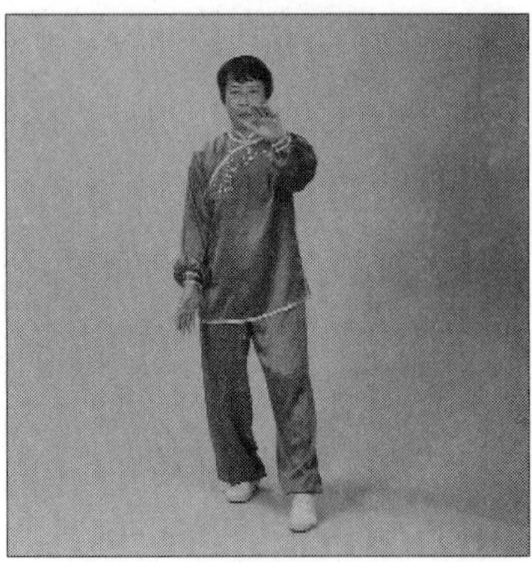

29 a. Turn the left palm down, and turn the right palm up. Fingers on both hands face forward.

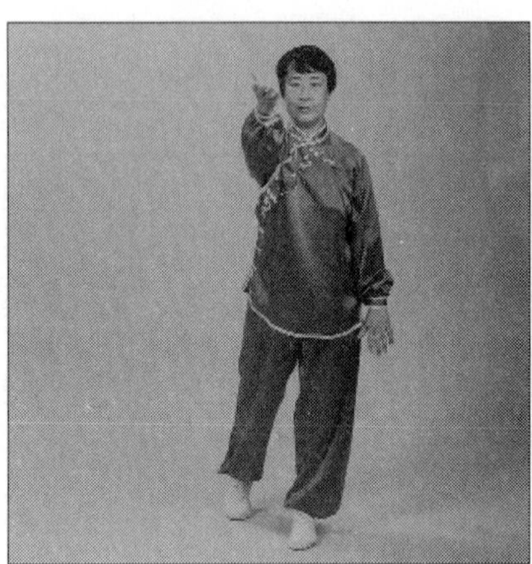

29 b-1. Gradually move the weight forward into the ball of the left foot, and raising both of the heels off the ground.While simultaneously bringing the right hand up to shoulder level and bringing the left hand down to hip level. Fingers on the right hand point forward, while fingers on the left hand point downward.

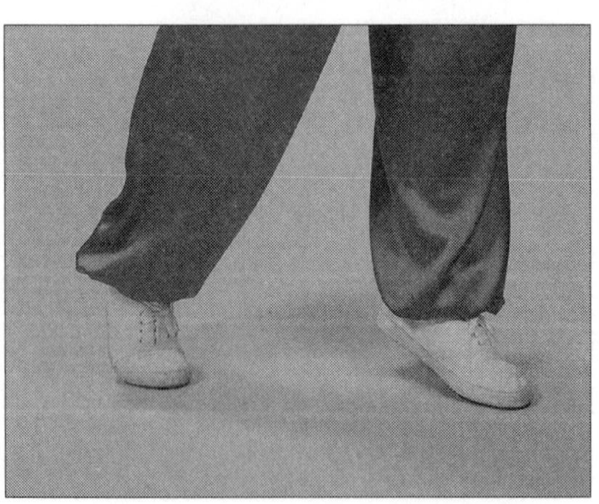

29 b-2. (ANOTHER ANGLE/CLOSE UP) The back right heel will probably raise higher than the forward left heel, because of the momentum of the body's weight being brought forward. Prepare for the Heels Down (Force) method.

CHI ESSENTIALS: Yang energy is gathered at the Laogong point as the right palm rises, while Yin energy is brought down as the left palm goes down. Refer to the basics covering the Rising and Falling Palms methods for more visuals and explanations.

30. RECOVER AIR

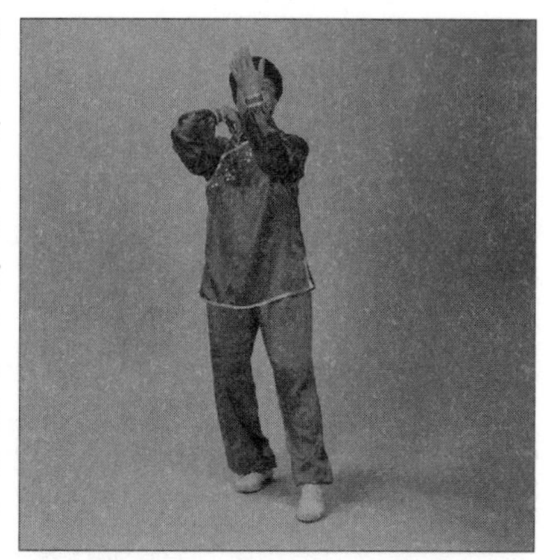

30 a-1. Utilizing the Heels Down (Force) method, bring the body's weight down into the right foot to assume the left Empty Stance (Ball of the Foot). Simultaneously, bring the Laogong point on the left hand to face the Upward Dantian at the Yintang point which is located between the eyebrows. While, the right hand forms the Eagle's Beak which points downward and contacts the right Quepen point which is located just above the right collar bone (vertically in line with the right nipple).

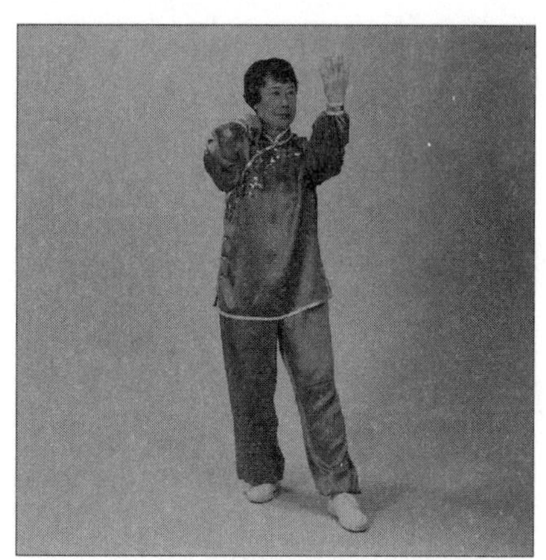

30 a-2. (ANOTHER ANGLE) Keep both shoulders relaxed, while the eyes focus on the Laogong point in the left palm, and the right Eagle's Beak contacts the right Quepen point.

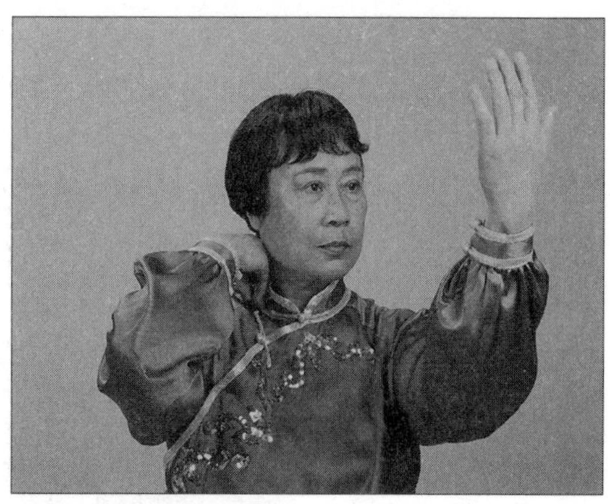

30 a-3. (ANOTHER ANGLE/CLOSE UP.) The fingers on the left hand point upward to the sky. The fingers on the right hand form the Eagle's Beak and point downward into the right Quepen point. The eyes focus on the left palm.

CHI ESSENTIALS: The right Eagle's Beak brings fresh Chi into the right Quepen point, which is located on the Stomach Channel. As the Chi comes down naturally through the chest, the Lung Channel is contacted and stimulated. While simultaneously the left palm pours fresh Chi in the Upward Dantian, which is ultimately brought down to the Lower Dantian for storage. The Heels Down (Force) method is used to shock the channels on the legs to bring the Yang energy up and the Yin energy down for dredging the channels on the legs of bad chi.

31. SCOOP THE MOON

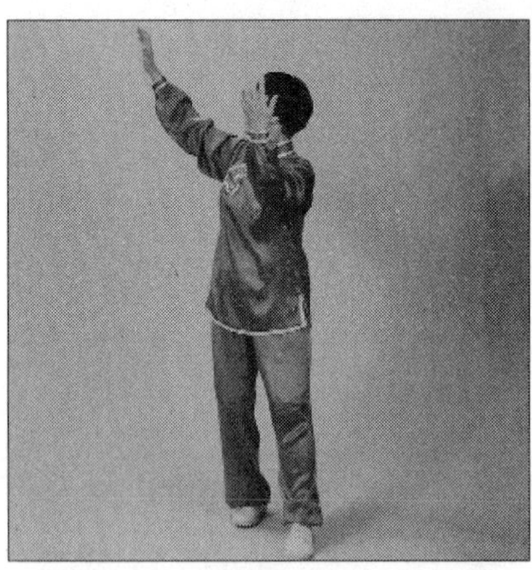

31 a-1. Turn the waist to the right, while bringing the right hand 135 degrees back right from the front. The right palm faces outward, and reaches upward. The eyes follow the back of the right hand. The left hand remains the same, as does the left Empty stance (Ball of the Foot).

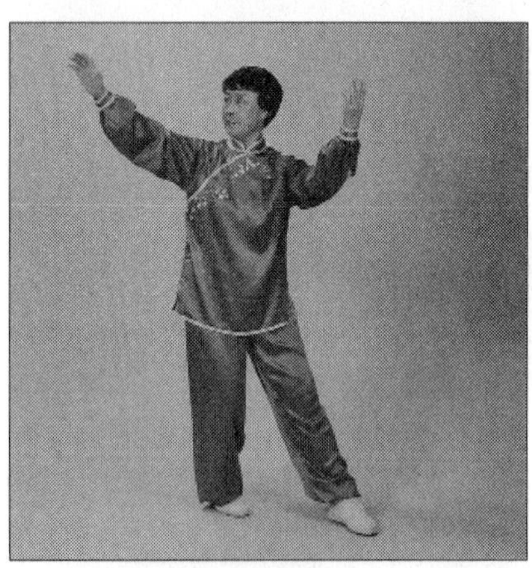

31 a-2. (ANOTHER ANGLE) The fingers on both hands point upward. The right palm faces outward and reaches upward. Eyes follow the back of the right hand. Left palm continues to face inward level with the Upward Dantian.

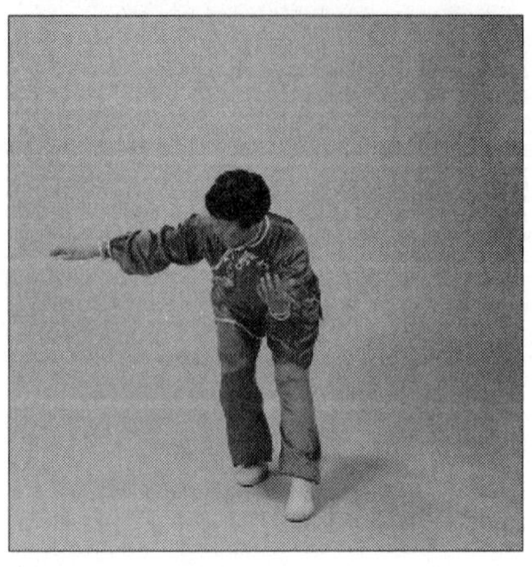

31 b. Gradually squat into the right leg, while bringing the right arm down. Palm faces down to the Earth. The left palm comes down as the body bends, but still remains level with the Upward Dantian.

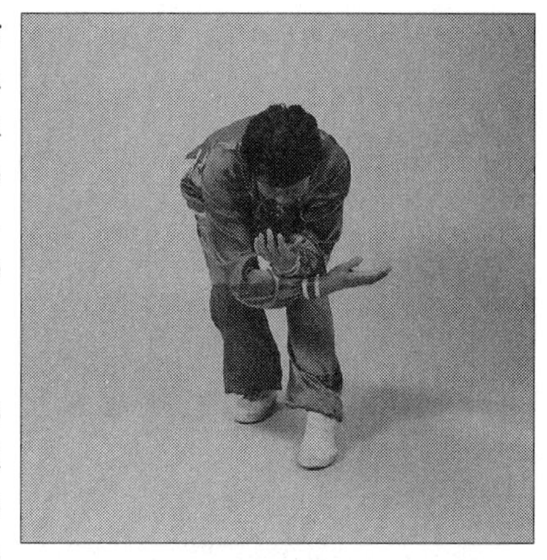

31 c. Continue squatting into the right leg gradually, while bringing the right palm down as far as possible until the fingers turn and point downward naturally towards the Earth. Then circle the right palm inward. Crossing horizontally the vertical line of the left arm. Look at the left palm.

CHI ESSENTIALS: As the waist turns right, the left palm continues facing inward and level with the Upward Dantian. Then the left palm faces the left ear, where Chi is poured in the left ear; stimulating and warming the Triple Warmer Channel. The right hand reaches outward and upward, gathering fresh Chi. As the right hand circles and continues gathering an enormous amount of Chi, the body bends forward. Bending of the body helps to bring the Chi down to the Lower Dantian to be stored.

32. TURN BODY

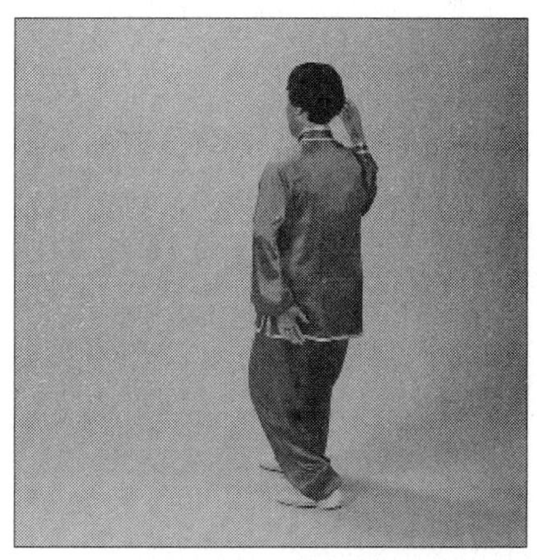

32 a-1. Gradually stand up, while turning the left toe inward 90-135 degrees. Then, while continuing to gradually stand up, turn the right toe out to the right and back 90-135 degrees. Let the left hand come down to the left side of the buttocks, and the right hand is level with the Upward Dantian. Look forward in the direction of the right toe.

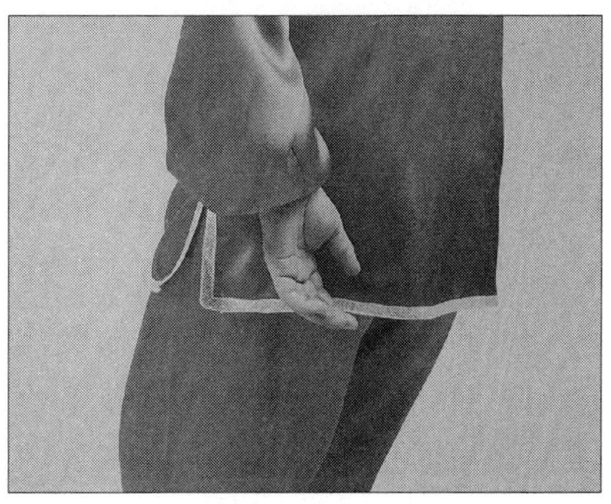

32 a-2. (CLOSE UP) The fingers on the left hand point downward. Making it easier for the Hegu point on the left hand to contact the Huantiao point on the left side of the buttocks.

CHI ESSENTIALS: When the body comes up pressure is felt at the Quepen and Qihu points stimulating the Stomach Channel. The Hegu point on the left hand contacts and stimulates the Gall Bladder Channel. The right hand is level with and contacting the Upward Dantian.

33. STEP FORWARD AND LOOK AT PALM

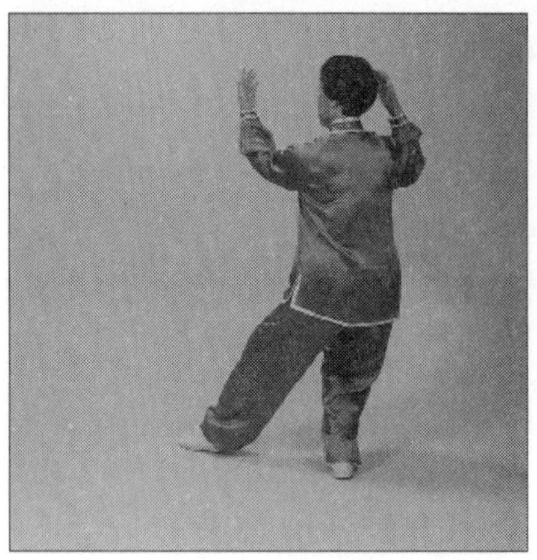

33-1. Turn the right toe outward to the right 45 degrees more. Gently extend the right foot forward, assuming the left Empty stance (Ball of the Foot). Simultaneously raise the left palm to face the Upward Dantian at the Yintang point, while turning the right elbow out slightly to raise the right hand to face the right temple. Look at the left palm.

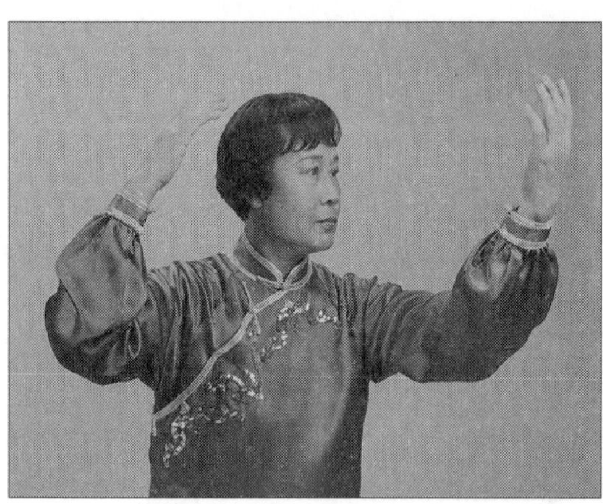

33-2. (REVERSE ANGLE/CLOSE UP) The fingers on both hands point upward. Relax the shoulders while the Laogong point on the left hand faces the Yintang point between the eyebrows, and the right palm faces the Taiyang point located at the left side of the head at the temple.

CHI ESSENTIALS: The right palm pours Chi into Upward Dantian by way of the Taiyang point. While the left hand pours Chi into the Upward Dantian by way of the Yintang point. This fresh Chi will ultimately drop down to be stored in the Lower Dantian.

34. LOOK UP TO THE MOON

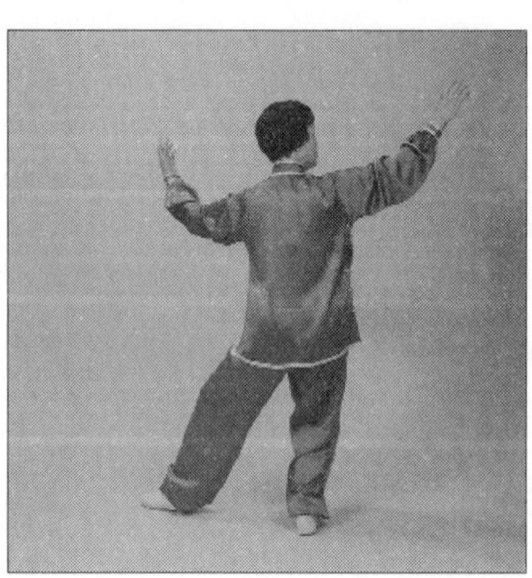

34 a. Turn the waist right, while bringing the right hand no more than 135 degrees back right from your current angle. The right palm faces outward, and reaches upward. The eyes follow the back of the right hand. The left hand remains level with the Upward Dantian, while the left Empty stance (Ball of the Foot) is maintained.

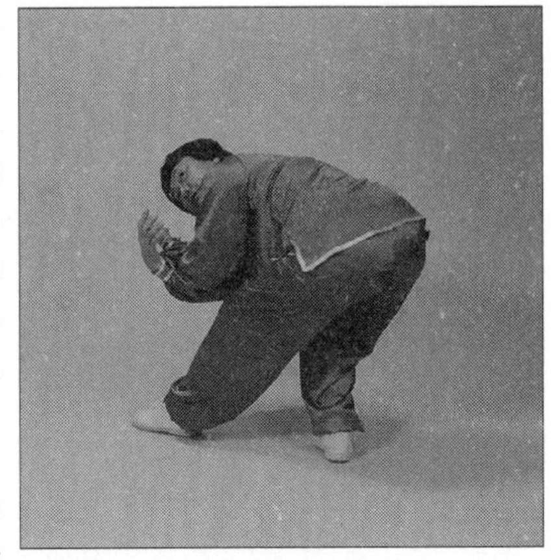

34 b. Suddenly swing the right arm downward, making a big circle, and drawing the right arm horizontally across the vertical line of the left arm. The inside of the right forearm comes up to firmly strike the outside of the left forearm. Relax the right hand, and let the wrist be loose to vibrate.The eyes follow the right hand around, and then look up to the sky.

CHI ESSENTIALS: As the waist turns the Dai Meridian works all the Yin and Yang Channels of the body. When the waist turns right, and the eyes follow the back of the right hand, the left palm pours Chi into the left ear for stimulating and warming the Triple Warmer Channel. The right hand reaches outward and upward, gathering fresh Chi. As the right arm swings down and gains momentum, bad chi is dredged. When the inside of the right forearm firmly strikes the outside of the left forearm, bad Chi is thrown out. That's why it's important here to bring the right palm outside the body more, relax the right hand, and let the right wrist be loose; in order that the right hand can vibrate and throw out all the bad chi. The movement forward and downward at the waist helps store Chi that was poured in the Upward Dantian from the previous form, Step Forward And Look At Palm. This movement helps to open and stimulate the left Urinary Bladder Channel and the right Gallbladder Channel, while simultaneously helping to cleanse the Urinary Bladder and Liver Channels of bad chi and helping to stimulate all the other channels of the body.

35. PRESS AIR

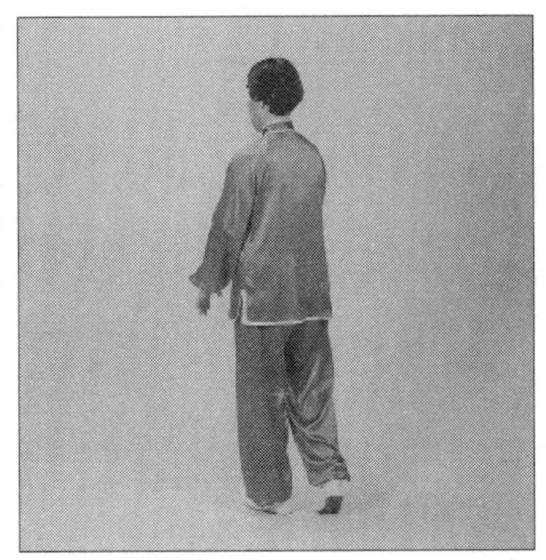

35 a. Gradually stand up, while bringing palms down, level with the pelvic region. Move the weight forward into the left foot, and the right foot takes a half a step forward onto the ball of the right foot. Raise right heel. The eyes look forward in the direction of the left toe on your current angle.

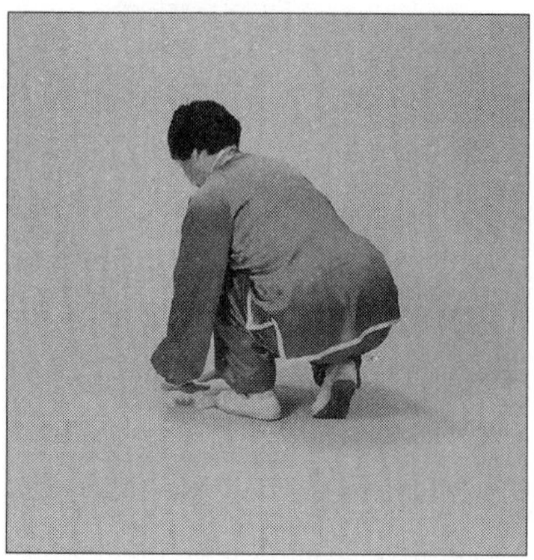

35 b-1. Gradually squat, and use the downward motion to help press palms downward towards the ground. The eyes look at the backs of the hands.

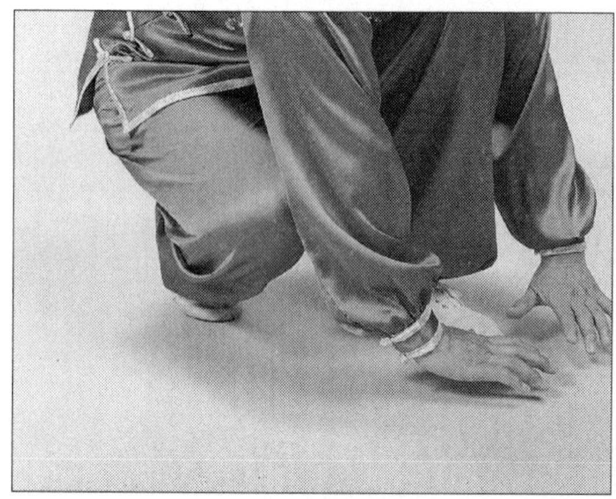

35 b-2. (REVERSE ANGLE/CLOSE UP) The fingers point inward towards each other slightly. The thumbs point towards each other. The palms press down in front of the left foot towards the ground, but don't touch.

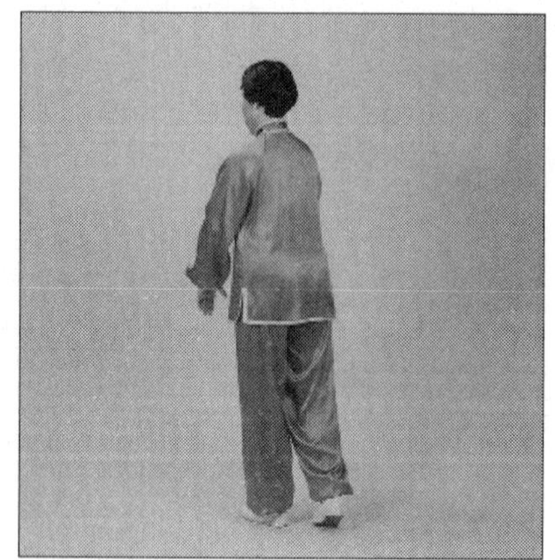

35 c. Gradually stand up, allowing the palms to gradually relax. The weight remains mostly in the left leg. The palms return to the lower pelvic region, palms face inward.

Repeat movements 35 b-1. and 35 c. two more times for a total of three repetitions.

CHI ESSENTIALS: The form helps to open and stimulate the Yin and Yang channels on the feet. When the body comes up, the hands relax opening the Laogong and the Yongquan point on the feet to receive Chi. When you press the palms downward and squat, Chi is encouraged to come down to be stored in the Lower Dantian. While bad chi is encouraged to come down, and be dispelled from the Yongquan point near the center of the ball of the foot and from the palms at the Laogong points. The stretching up and down helps strengthen joints, muscles, and connective tissue on the legs; as well as relieving lower back pain. Furthermore, the stretching up and down strengthens the stomach and intestines.

36. TURN BODY AND PRESS AIR

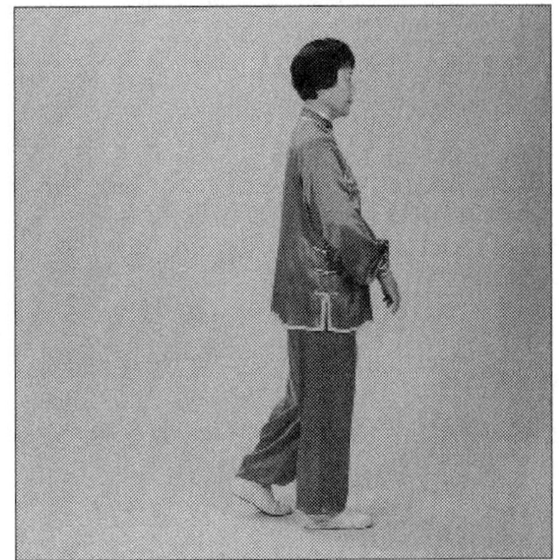

36 a. The hands stay level with the lower pelvic region, palms facing inward. Then on the balls of the feet pivot 135 degrees to the right. The right foot is in front facing a new angle, and the left is behind the right foot with the toes on the left facing outward 45 degrees left with the new direction.

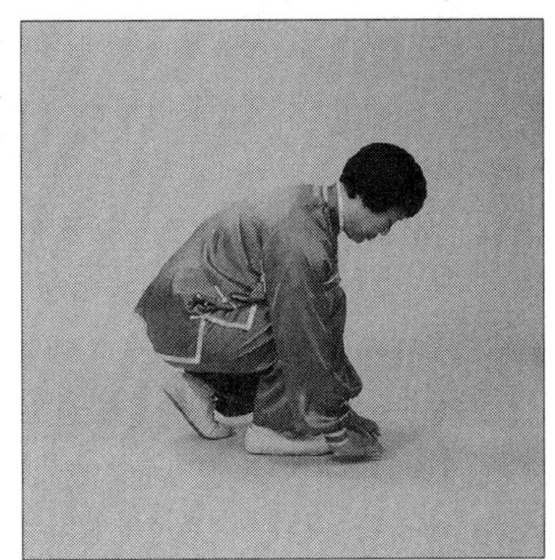

36 b-1. Then as in movement 35 b-1., gradually squat, and press palms downward towards the ground. The eyes look at the backs of the hands.

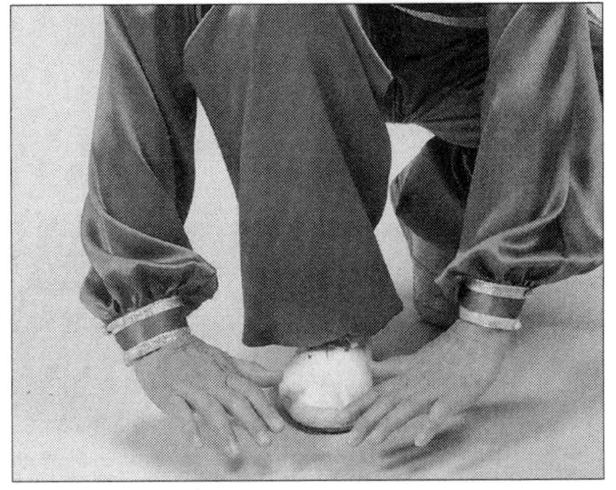

36 b-2. (ANOTHER ANGLE/CLOSE UP) The fingers point inward towards each other slightly. The thumbs point towards each other. The palms press down in front of the right foot towards the ground, but don't touch.

Repeat movements 36 a. and 36 b-1. two more times for a total of three repetitions.

CHI ESSENTIALS: See Chi Essentials for Form 35: Press Air.

37. SWIM FORWARD

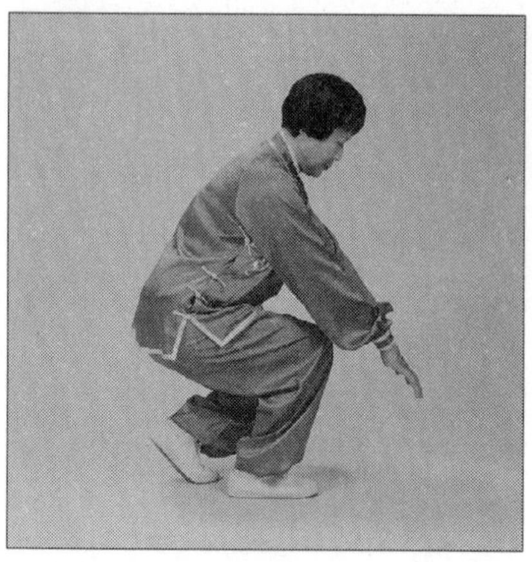

37 a. Gradually stand up with the weight in the right leg with the left heel raised, while extending both arms out and up with Shaking Palms. The Continuous Shaking Palms face downward.

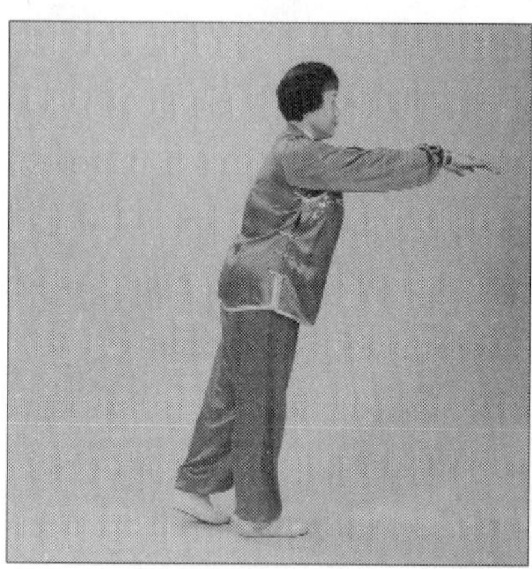

37 b. The left heel remains up, move the weight forward into the ball of the right foot, while continuing to extend the arms with Shaking Palms upward. The Continuous Shaking Palms still face downward all the way to shoulder level.

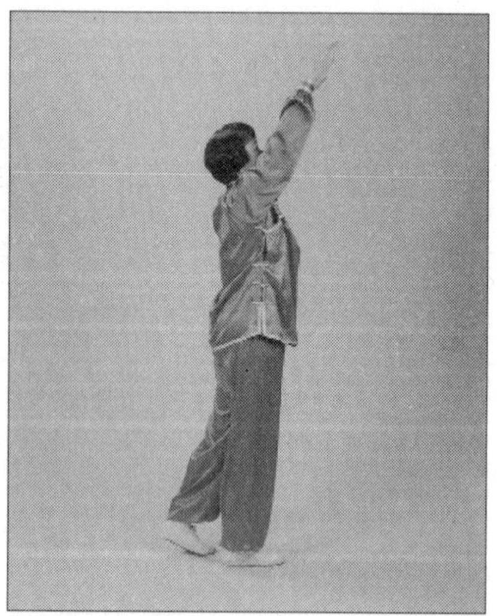

37 c. Continue raising and extending the Shaking Palms upward towards the sky. The Continuous Shaking Palms face outward.

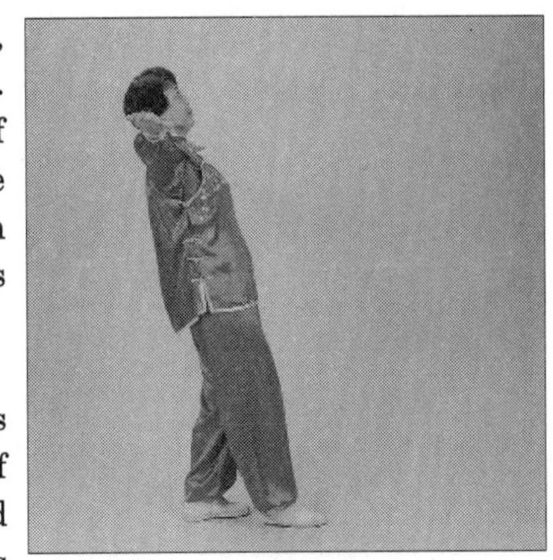

37 d. Shift the weight back in the left leg, and raise the right heel off the ground. Assuming the right Empty stance (Ball of the Foot). Simultaneously extend the Shaking Palms outward, bringing them gradually to shoulder level. The Continuous Shaking Palms face downward.

CHI ESSENTIALS: The Shaking Hands are accomplished by vibrating the bridge of the palm (at the base of the fingers), and allowing the arms and fingers to vibrate as well. By shaking the hands with moving the weight forward to extend out and up, and moving the weight back with continuous shaking of the hands, all 12 channels are opened and stimulated. The flow of blood and Chi is sped up and increased. The form also strengthens the internal energy.

38. LOOK DOWN AT WATER

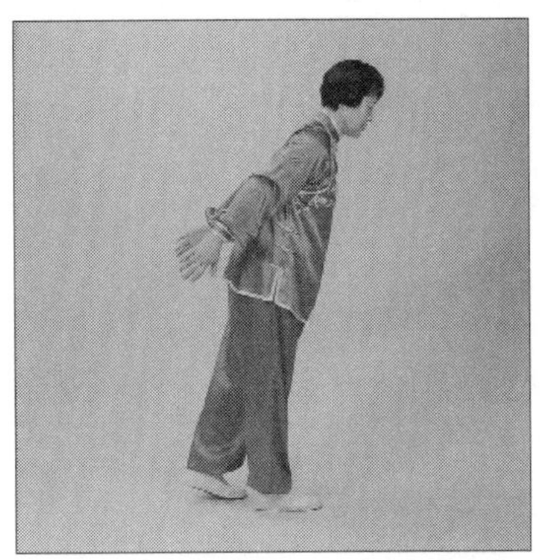

38-1. Gradually shift the weight forward onto the right foot and lift the left heel up. Continue Shaking Palms, and bring the palms behind you; level with the Sacrum. The eyes look out and downward on an angle toward the Earth. Continue Shaking Palms.

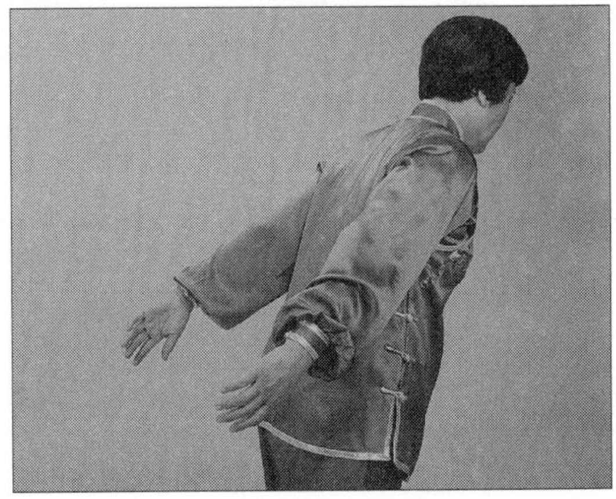

38-2. (ANOTHER ANGLE/CLOSE UP) The fingers on both of the hands point back and downward, behind the body, and level with the Sacrum. The Continuous Shaking Palms face each other. Continue shaking and relax in this posture momentarily.

CHI ESSENTIALS: The eyes, looking out and downward towards the ground, absorb the Earth's energy (Yin). As the Shaking Palms come back behind the body, level with the Sacrum, the Pericardium Channel is stimulated and the bad chi comes out through the fingers and palms.

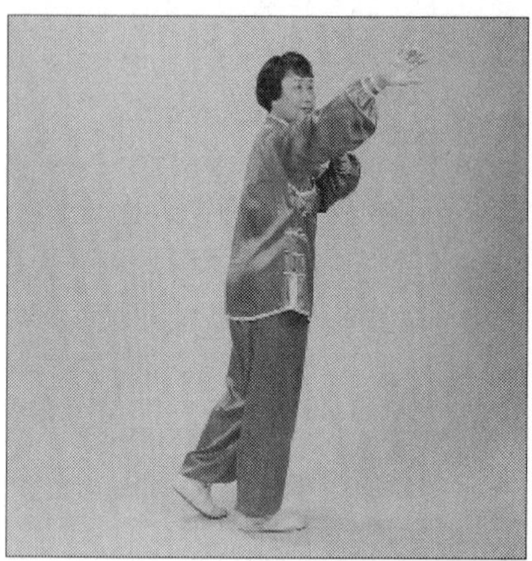

39. PAT WATER AND FLY AWAY

39 a-1. TRANSITION With the weight on the right foot and the left heel up, bring the Continuous Shaking Palms gradually in a curve forward and upward to the right. Simultaneously, the waist turns right, and the body stands more erect.

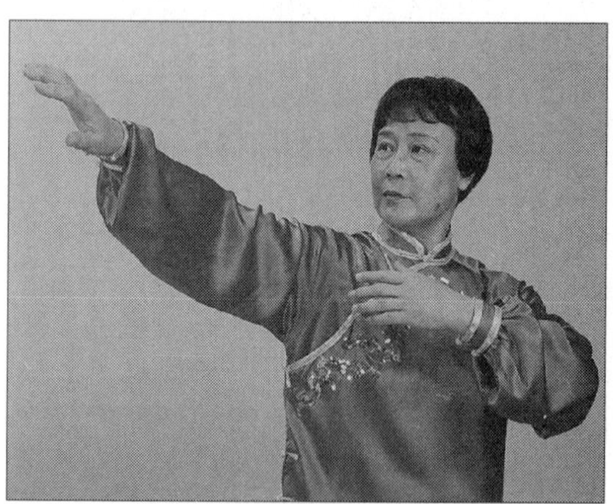

39 a-2. (ANOTHER ANGLE/CLOSE UP) The fingers on both continually shaking hands point away from the body's right side. The right palm faces outward and upward, while the Laogong point on the left palm faces the right Qihu point. The Qihu point is located below the right collar bone, and vertically aligned with the right nipple. The eyes look at the right hand.

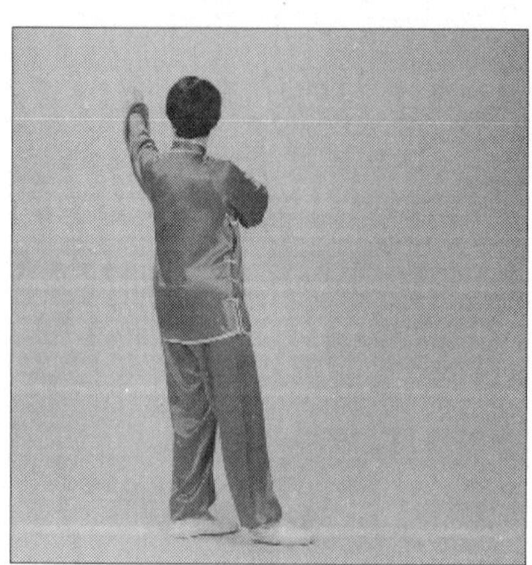

39 b-1. PAT WATER LEFT Then gradually turn the waist left, while bringing the Continuous Shaking Palms to the left. Simultaneously, shift the weight back into the left foot.

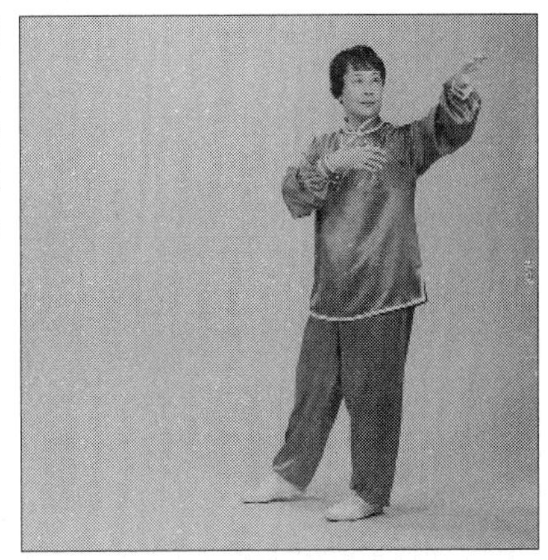

39 b-2. PAT WATER LEFT (REVERSE ANGLE) The fingers on both continually shaking hands point away from the body's left side. The left hand faces outward and upward, while the Laogong point on the right palm faces the left Qihu point.

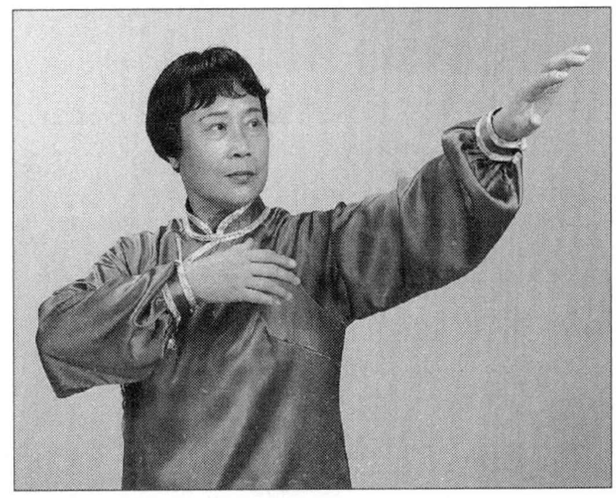

39 b-3. PAT WATER LEFT (REVERSE ANGLE/CLOSE UP) The shoulders should remain relaxed. Although the hands are continually shaking, the right hand is drawn in, and the left hand is extended outward and upward. The eyes look at the left hand.

Repeat movements 39 a-1. (which, when done again, is known as Pat Water Right) and 39 b-1 (Pat Water Left) one more time. So the sequence after the transition (39 a-1 done the first time) is Pat Water Left, Right, and Left.

CHI ESSENTIALS: Moving the hand, feet, waist, and back at the same time opens the Dai and Du meridians simultaneously. When the Laogong point continues shaking and moves outward and upward fresh Chi is gathered on the Laogong point of the palm. When the palm turns and comes inward and faces the Qihu point, fresh Chi is poured into the Qihu from the Laogong, and brought down to the Lower Dantian and Yongquan point with the movements of the weight shifting back and forth. As the weight moves back and forth together with the movement of the upper limbs, the soles of the feet rock back and forth to open all the channels on the feet.

40. DRINK WATER (3 X)

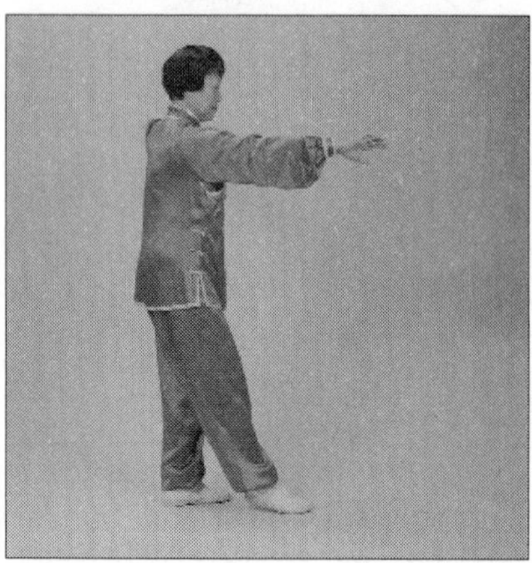

40 a. Upon completing the second Pat Water Left (see 39 b-1) turn the right heel inward, while horizontally circling the right Continuous Shaking Palm outward.

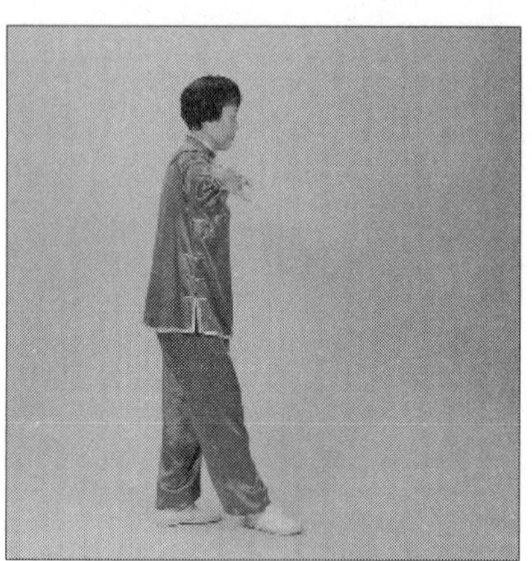

40 b. The Continuous Shaking Palms are both extended outward at shoulder level.

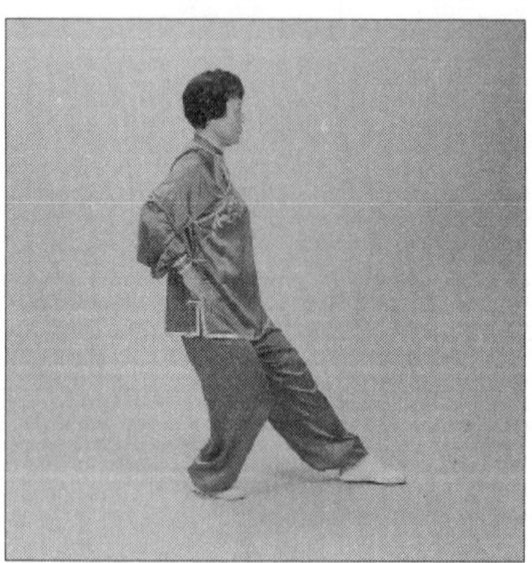

40 c. Gradually squat into the right leg, while gently extending the left foot outward. Assuming a slightly elongated left Empty stance (Ball of the Foot). Simultaneously both of the Continuous Shaking Palms are drawn inward on both sides of the waist. The palms face downward towards the Earth. Fingers, on both shaking hands, face slightly downward.

40 d. While keeping the torso straight, bend forward at the waist, and squat deeper into the right leg.

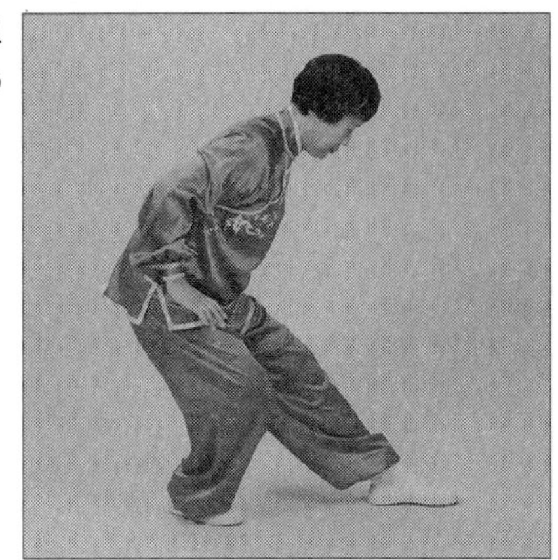

40 e. Both Continuous Shaking Palms move downward. The palms travel on parallel lines with the left palm tracing the outside of the left leg, and the right palm tracing the inside of the left leg, continuing through the left ankle.

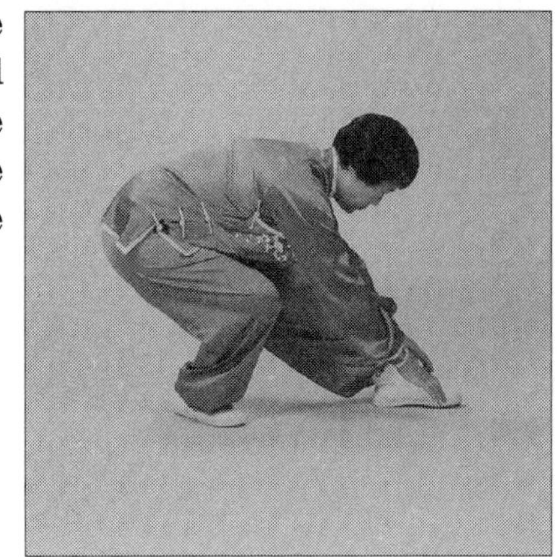

40 f. Gradually come up slightly and bring the Continuous Shaking Palms up.

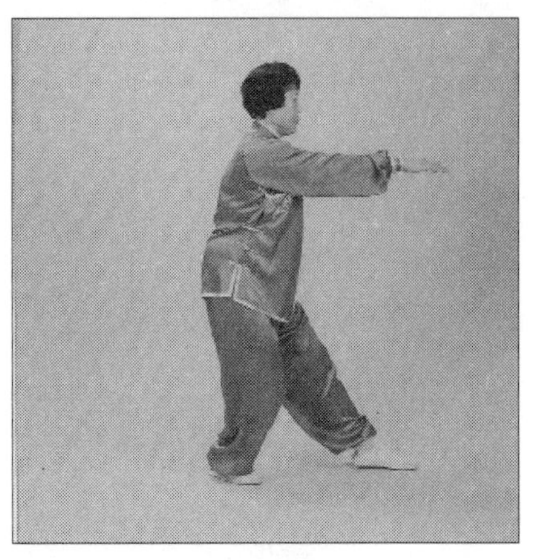

*Bring the Continuous Shaking Palms back to both sides of the waist, and repeat forms 40 c. through 40 f. two more times for a total of three repetitions.

CHI ESSENTIALS: The Qi comes in through the Baihui, Upward Dantian, and Yintang points. From there the Chi circulates two ways: 1) The Chi circulates from head to toe three times with the up and down movements. 2) The Pulmonary Circulation (small orbit) is encouraged on the Du and Ren Meridians three times as the vibrating limbs circle downward, upward, outward, and inward three times.

41. GAZE AT THE SKY

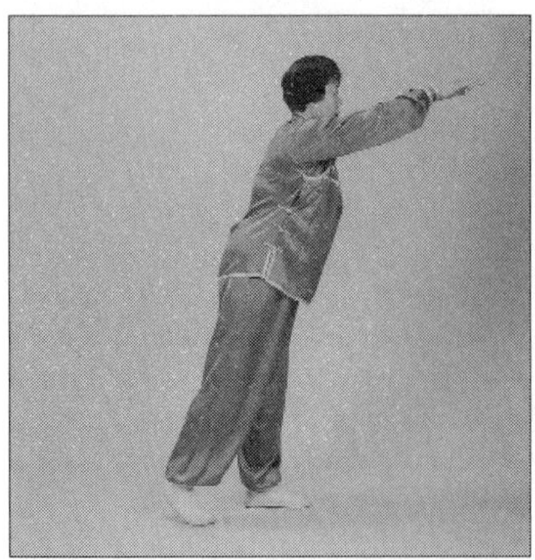

41 a. After the third time of Drink Water (see Form 40 f.) continue gradually coming up, extend and raise the Continuous Shaking Palms upward. Simultaneously, move the weight forward into the left foot, and raise the right heel off the ground as you bring the right foot forward slightly to maintain balance. Watch the Continuous Shaking Palms.

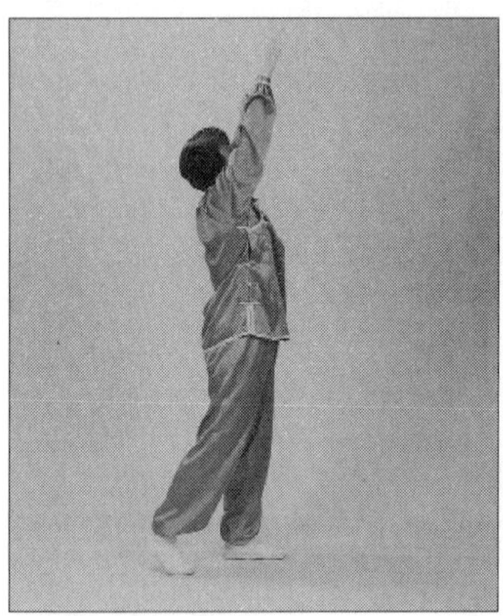

41 b. Continue extending the Continuous Shaking Palms upward, while eyes continue to follow the Shaking Palms upward. Gaze up at the sky.

CHI ESSENTIALS: When the two Shaking Palms extend outward and upward fresh Chi is gathered at the Laogong points on both hands. When the Shaking Palms extend upward, allow the Chi to come down and pass through the elbows, shoulders, and to the Qihu points on both sides of the body to be ultimately stored in the Lower Dantian.

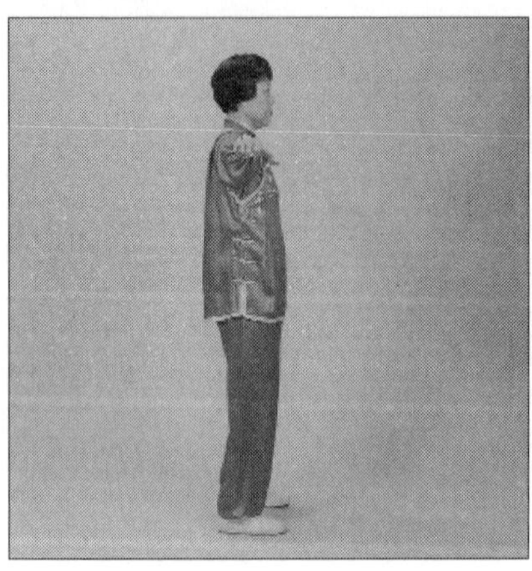

42. RECOVER AIR

42 a. Bring the Continually Shaking Palms down to shoulder level, palms facing down to the Earth. Simultaneously, bring the right foot forward, and assume a Parallel stance. When the palms reach shoulder level, the palms stop shaking, and pause momentarily. Meanwhile, the right foot should be finished moving forward, forming a Parallel stance.

42 b-1. Slowly bring the palms down and place them on the abdomen.

*Gently inhale deeply, and exhale softly. When the end of the exhale is reached, vibrate the palms on the abdomen vigorously. Try not to hold tightness in the wrists when shaking the palms. Repeat the breathing and vibrating of the palms two more times for a total of three times.

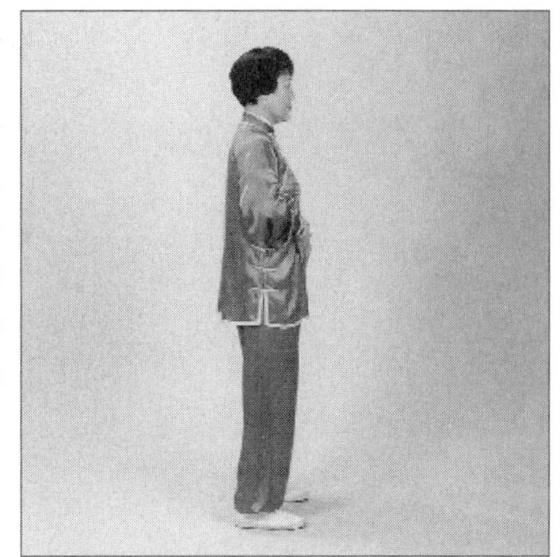

42 b-2. (ANOTHER ANGLE/CLOSE UP) This is the way the hands are traditionally placed on the abdomen for women. The tip of the right thumb is placed in the Shenque (Navel) point, pointing up through the Hegu point on the left hand which is placed above the right hand. The hands here form a Yin/Yang symbol.

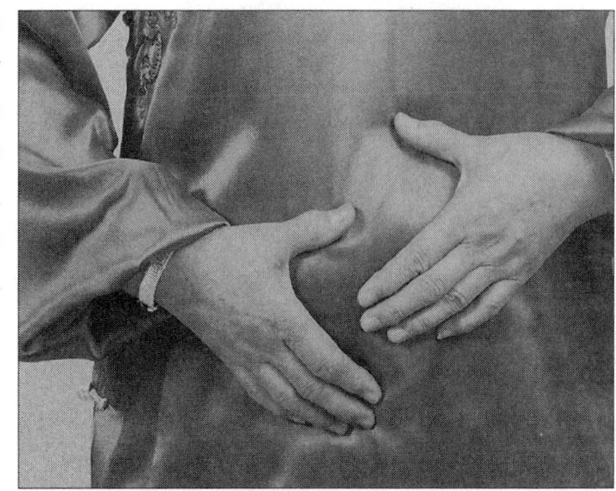

42 b-3. (ANOTHER ANGLE/CLOSE UP) This is the way the hands are traditionally placed on the abdomen for men. The tip of the left thumb is placed in the Shenque (Navel) point, pointing up through the Hegu point on the right hand which is placed above the left hand. Again the hand placement forms a Yin/Yang symbol.

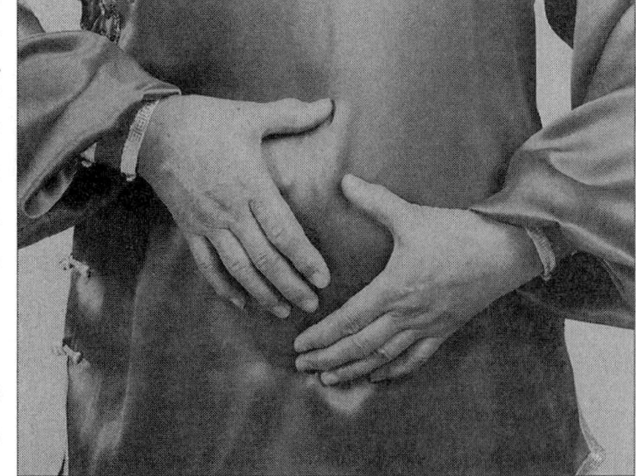

CHI ESSENTIALS: When the two hands spread out to shoulder level and then come in and down to the abdomen, Chi is naturally brought down to the Lower Dantian from the Upward Dantian, through the Middle Dantian, and from the Qihu point collected from the previous form: Gaze at the Sky. Also the stomach channel is stimulated when the two hands are placed on both sides of the navel, and the palms vibrate three times.

43. GRASP AIR

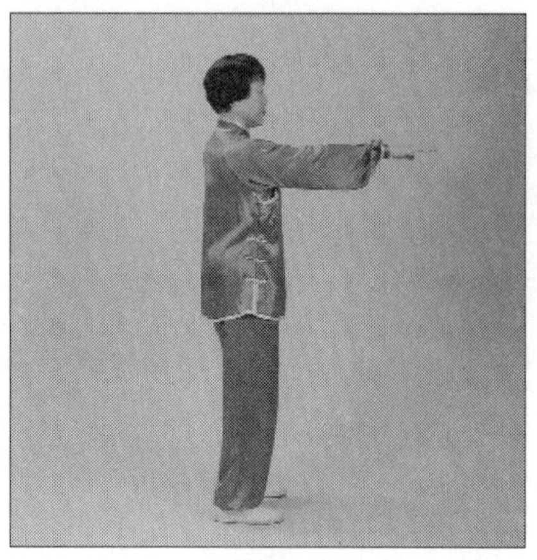

43 a. Raise right hand out and extend forward to your current direction of practice. Palm faces downward toward the Earth. Then bring the right palm inward, gradually forming a right hollow fist. Bring the right hollow fist in below the right clavicle with the thumb and forefinger of the right hollow fist resting against the body. The palm side of the right hollow fist faces toward the Earth. If you were to take your left forefinger and bring it through the center of the hollow fist to touch the body, the tip of the left finger should be touching your right Qihu point (located below the right clavicle, vertically aligned with the right nipple). The right elbow is on the same horizontal line as the right hollow fist. The left hand remains placed on the abdomen from the previous form.

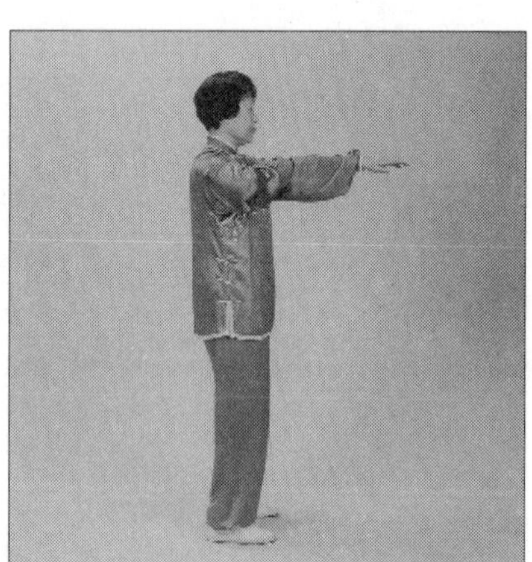

43 b-1. Then raise and extend the left hand out forward to your current direction of practice. Palm faces downward toward the Earth. Then bring the left palm inward, gradually forming a left hollow fist. Bring the left hollow fist in below the left clavicle with the thumb and forefinger of the left hollow fist resting against the body.

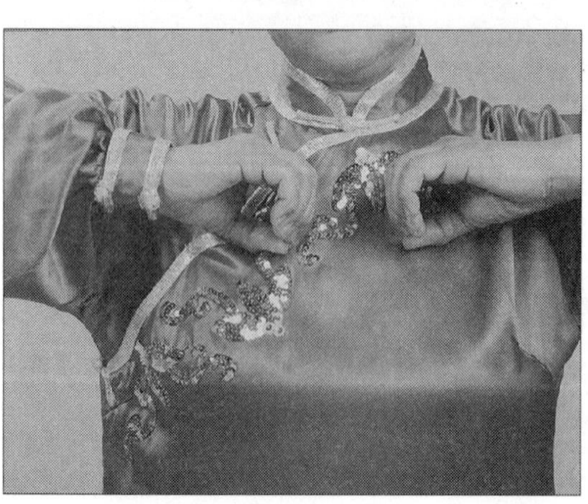

43 b-2. (ANOTHER ANGLE/CLOSE UP) This shows the position of both hollowed fists after the second repetition. The form, Grasp Air, is to be done a total of ten times.

As you can see if you were to place a finger through either hollow fist to touch the body, the tip of the probing finger would contact the Qihu point (located below the clavicles, and vertically aligned with the nipples) which is located on both sides of the body. Furthermore, the elbows share the same horizontal line as the hollow fists. While the elbows are raised, do not raise the shoulders up. Keep your shoulders down and relaxed.

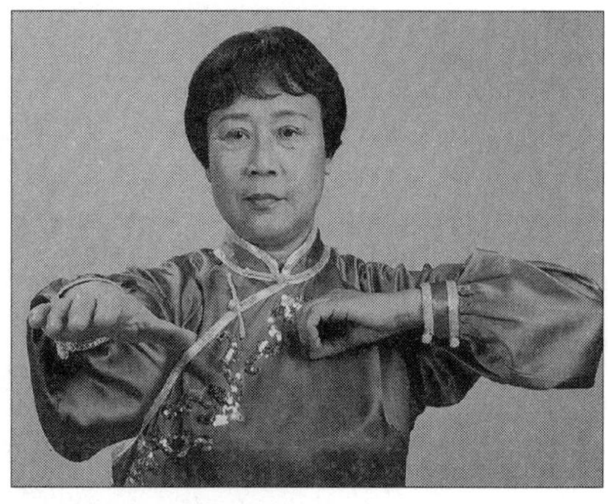

43 c. (ANOTHER ANGLE/CLOSE UP) As you continue to begin the third repetition, extend the right hand forward. Palm faces downward towards the Earth. Notice as you extend the hand forward the space between the thumb and forefinger is open and rounded. The left hollow fist remains on the body with the center of the left hollow fist surrounding the left Qihu point. Furthermore, notice that the left elbow remains on the same horizontal line as the left hollow fist without raised or tightened up shoulders.

Then bring the right palm in gradually changing it into a right hollow fist. Bringing the right hollow fist in, so that the right forefinger and thumb rest on the chest below the right clavicle (See 43 b-2).

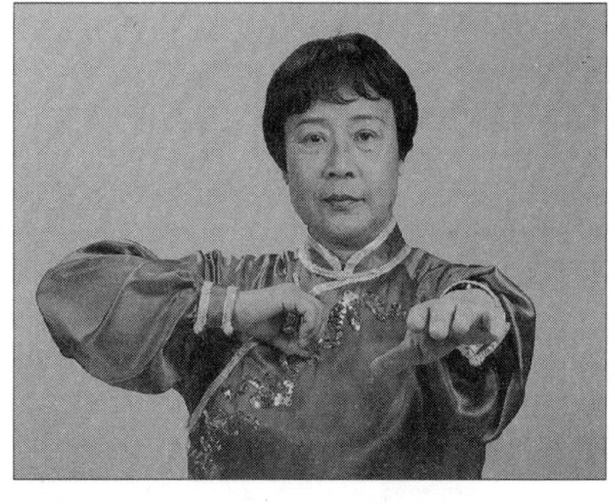

43 d. (ANOTHER ANGLE/CLOSE UP) As you continue to do the fourth repetition, extend the left hand forward. Palm faces downward towards the Earth. Notice again, the roundness of the space between the thumb and forefinger. The right hollow fist remains on the body with the center of the right hollow fist surrounding the right Qihu point. Furthermore, notice that the right elbow remains on the same horizontal line as the right hollow fist without raised or tightened up shoulders.

*After you bring the left hand inward to place the hollow fist on the body below the left collar bone (See 43 b-2), you will have completed a total of four repetitions. Then repeat movements 43 c, 43 b-2, 43 d, and 43 b-2 in that order. Extending each hand forward and bringing in the hollow fist six more times for a total of ten repetitions.

CHI ESSENTIALS: Grasp fresh air from nature, when the Yin (Faces Earth) palm extends forward, and then gradually changes to the hollow fist. Coming back to rest against the body. The relaxed palm that extends forward, keeping the space between the thumb and forefinger opened, will naturally open the Hegu point on the hand. In the Hegu point receive the Chi from nature and bring the hollow fist to store this fresh Chi in the Qihu point (located below the clavicle, aligned vertically with the nipple). From there allow the fresh Chi to sink to the Lower Dantian, while you continue to grasp more fresh Chi from nature.

44. TURN UP PALM AND GATHER UP AIR

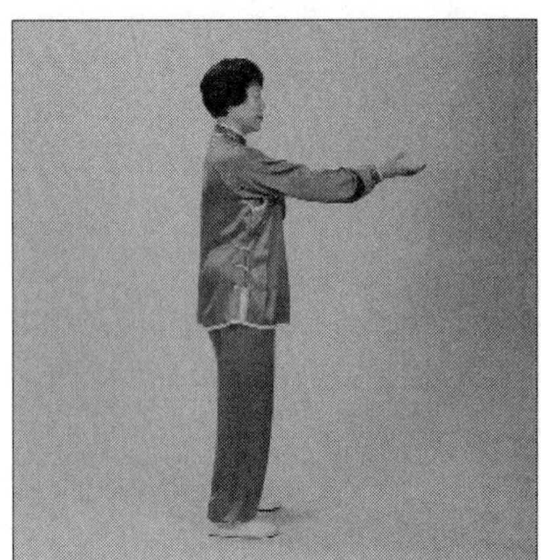

44 a. With the left hollow fist still surrounding the left Qihu point and the left elbow up sharing the same horizontal line as the left hollow fist, extend the right hand forward to shoulder level. The right palm faces upward toward the sky. Then bring the right Yang palm in, gradually changing into a right hollow fist, to the right side of the chest below the clavicle. The small finger of the right hollow fist rests on the chest, while the palm of the right hollow fist faces upward.

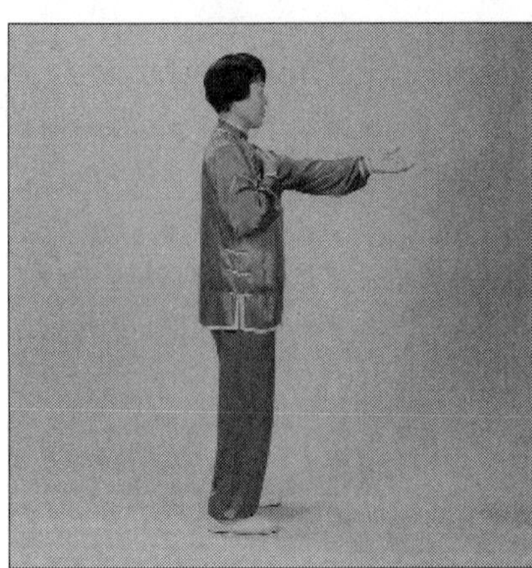

44 b-1. Extend the left hand forward to shoulder level. The palm faces upward toward the sky. Then bring the left Yang palm in, gradually changing into a left hollow fist. Bring the left hollow fist in to the left side of the chest below the left clavicle with the small finger of the left hollow fist resting against the body.

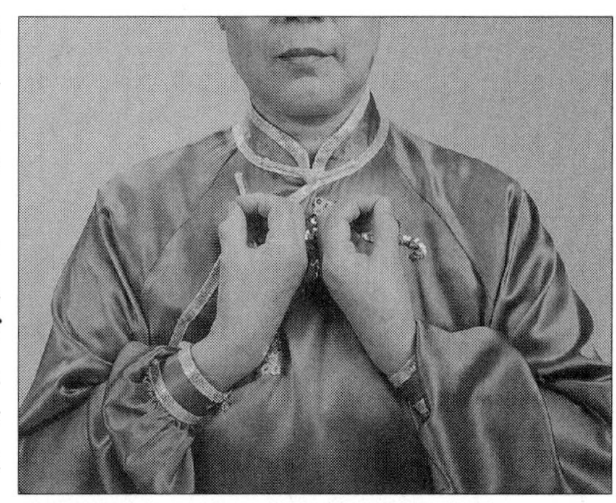

44 b-2. (ANOTHER ANGLE/CLOSE UP) This shows the position of both hollowed fists after the second repetition. The form, Turn Up Palm and Gather Up Air, is to be done a total of ten times.

Again, as in the previous form, Grasp Air, if you were to place a finger through either hollow fist to touch the body, the tip of the probing finger would contact the Qihu point (located below the clavicle, vertically aligned with the nipple) which is located on both sides of the body.

Different with the previous form are the elbows which are downward with the tips of the elbows pointing towards the Earth.

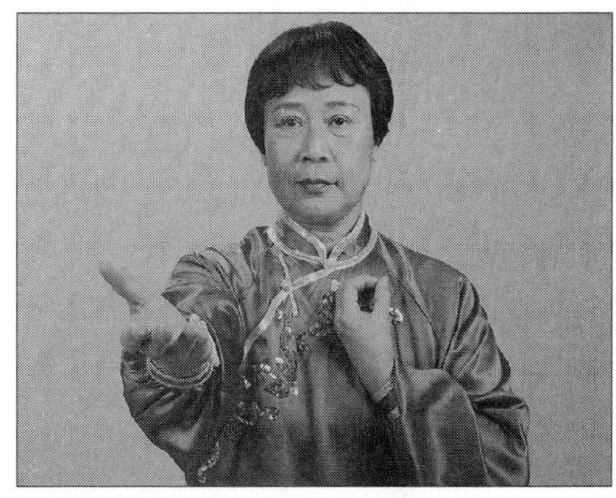

44 c. (ANOTHER ANGLE/CLOSE UP) As you continue to begin to do the third repetition extend the right hand forward. Palm faces upward towards the sky. Notice as you extend the hand forward the space between the thumb and forefinger is open and rounded. The left hollow fist remains on the body with the center of the left hollow fist surrounding the left Qihu point. Furthermore, notice that the left elbow remains pointing downward toward the Earth. Notice also that the shoulders do not raise or tighten up.

Then bring the right turned up palm in gradually changing into a right hollow fist. Bringing the right hollow fist in, so that the small finger on the right hollow fist rests on the chest below the right clavicle (See 44 b-2).

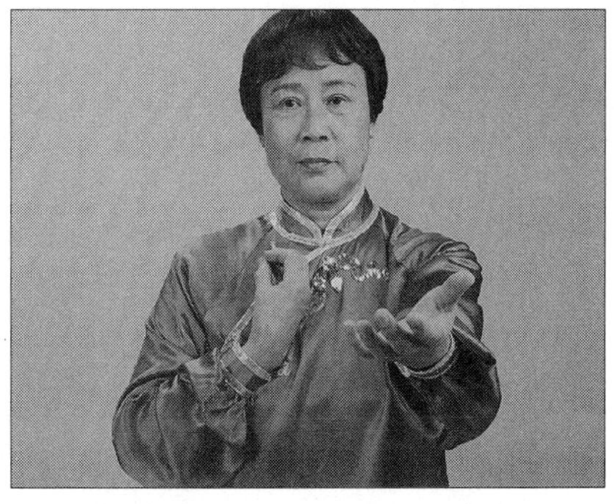

44 d. (ANOTHER ANGLE/CLOSE UP) As you continue to do the fourth repetition, extend the left hand forward. Palm faces upward towards the sky. Notice again, the roundness of the space between the thumb and forefinger. The right hollow fist remains on the body with the center of the hollow fist surrounding the right Qihu point. Furthermore, notice that the right elbow points downward towards the Earth.

*After you bring the left hand inward to place the hollow fist on the body below the left collar bone (See 43 b-2), you will have completed four repetitions. Then repeat movements 44 c, 44 b-2, 44 d, and 44 b-2 in that order. Extending each hand forward and bringing in the hollow fist six more times for a total of ten repetitions.

CHI ESSENTIALS: Again like form 43, Grasp Air, you are extending the palm outward and gradually changing the palm into a hollow fist for the purpose of gathering fresh Chi to place in the Qihu point. Then as you continue gathering the Chi, you sink the Chi into the Lower Dantian for storage. The Qihu (or, Chi Door) is one of the major points of Wild Goose Chi Kung practice. This form, as well as the previous one, help to open and stimulate the Qihu. This in turn helps to relax the chest, regulate the flow of vital energy, and remove any obstructions on all twelve channels.

45. HOLD BALL

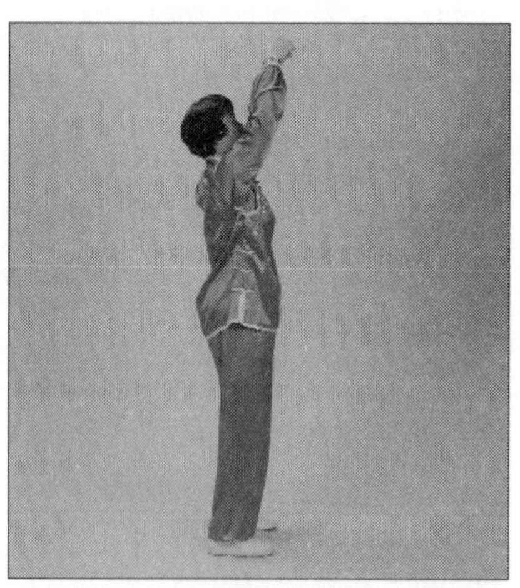

45 a. Release the hollow fists that are both resting on the chest, change the hollow fists to palms, and extend both palms upward towards the sky. Eyes look up at the hands.

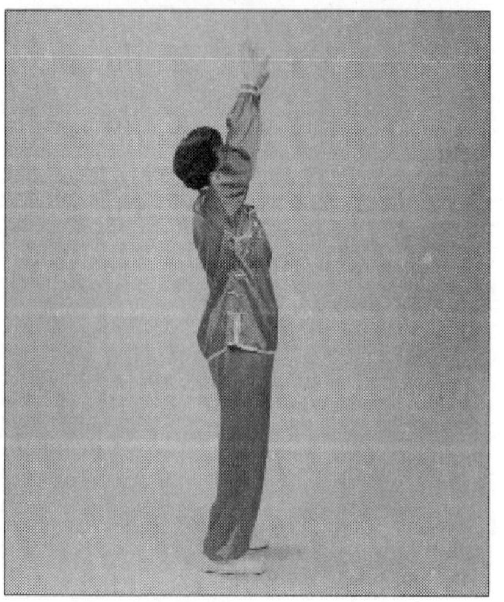

45 b. Then, turn the palms outward.

45 c. Then while gradually bending forward at the waist, let the hands come outward and downward on a curve. Let the palms naturally turn inwards.

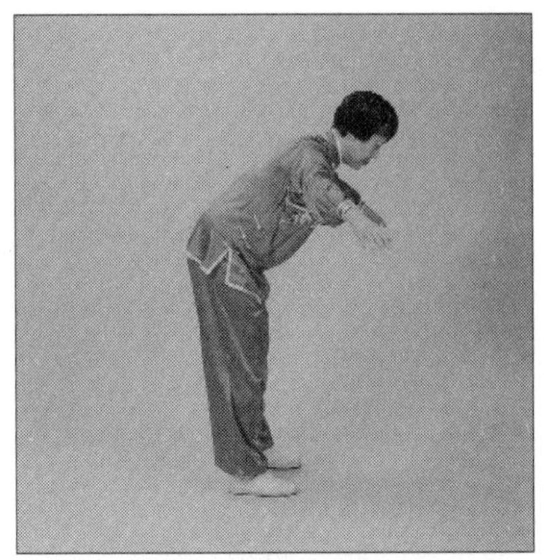

45 d. Continue bending over, if possible, and let the arms be rounded as if holding a ball between your arms. Remember to not bend your head lower than your heart if you have high blood pressure or heart problems. Also do not bend your knees to go down farther. Keep your legs locked, and go down as far as you can. The eyes look down at the palms, and keep your neck relaxed.

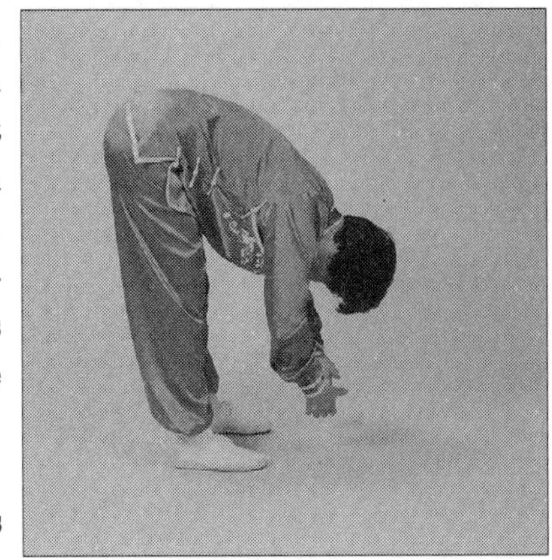

CHI ESSENTIALS: Raising the arms upward opens and stimulates the three Yin channels of the hands. When bending at the waist and the arms come down, the three Yang channels of the hands are opened and stimulated. When the two arms embrace an imaginary ball, a large ball of fresh Chi is gathered.

46. ROTATE THE BALL

46 a. Lift up the torso slightly, while still holding an imaginary ball between the arms.

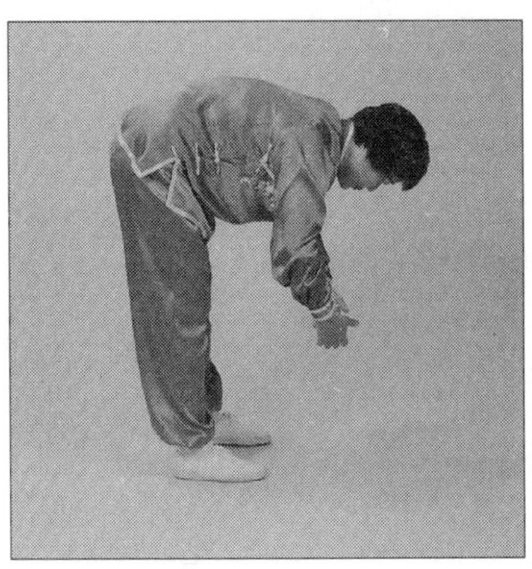

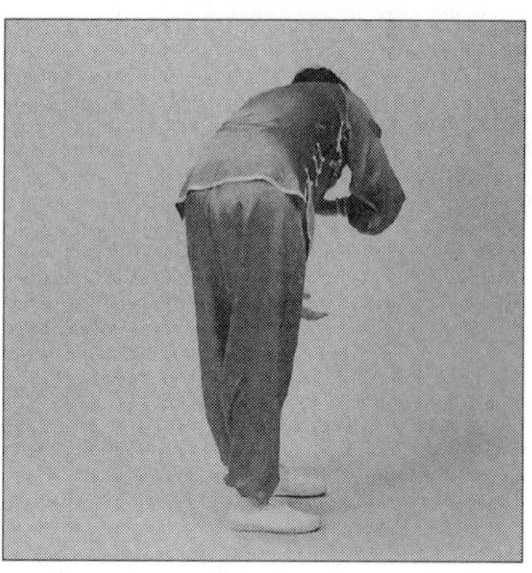

46 b-1. Gently turn with waist to the left, while maintaining holding an imaginary ball between the arms. Then bring the right palm above to face down at the left palm. Look at the hands.

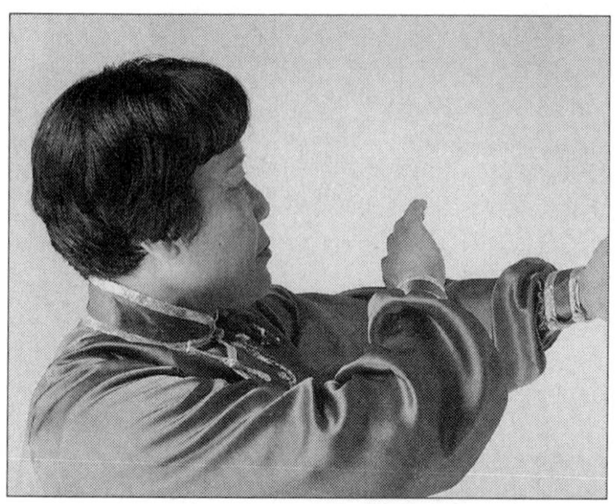

46 b-2. (ANOTHER ANGLE/CLOSE UP) The right palm faces directly over and down towards the left palm. Between the two palms is an imaginary ball. Then begin gradually turning with the waist to the right. As you do so, wiggle all the fingers on both hands. Simultaneously, circle the top hand inward (bringing in fresh Chi), and circle the bottom hand outward (bringing out bad chi).

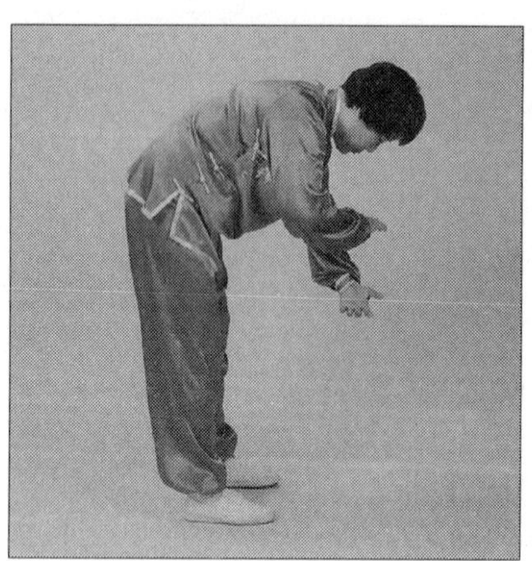

46 c-1. It should take to the count of five to return to the center where you began. Continue turning with the waist to the right, wiggling the fingers, while circling the top hand inward, and the bottom hand outward.

46 c-2. (ANOTHER ANGLE/CLOSE UP) Again, it should take five counts to reach the center. There is a total of ten counts to reach the right side, and there the palms change.

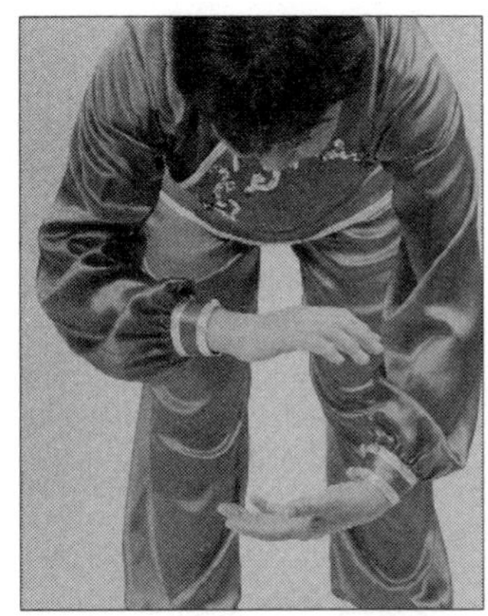

46 d-1. Continue turning the waist to the right, wiggling the fingers, while circling the top hand inward and the bottom hand outward. All the way to the right side.

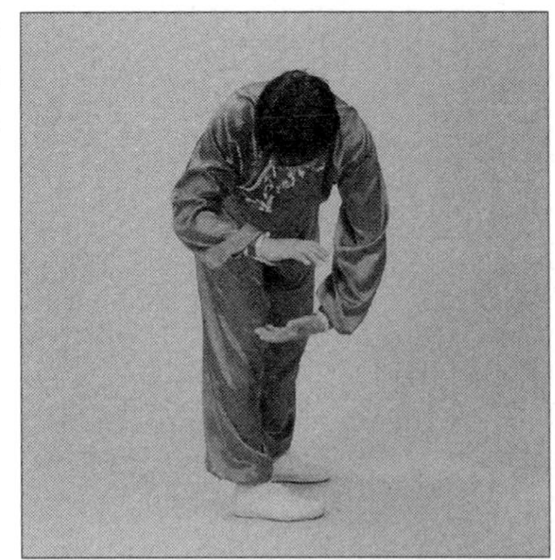

46 d-2. (ANOTHER ANGLE/CLOSE UP) By the tenth count, you should be turned all the way to the right side.

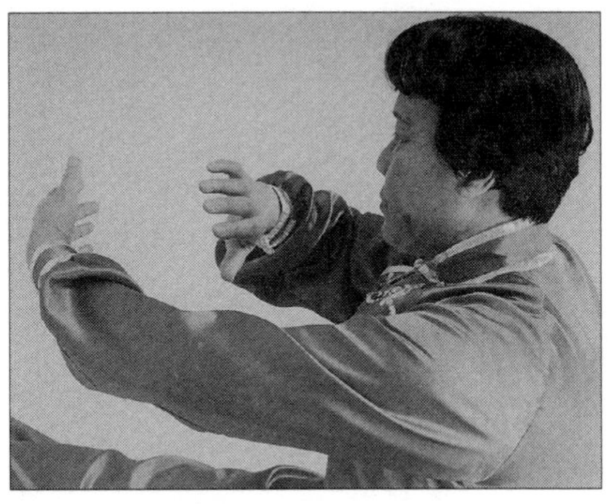

CHI ESSENTIALS: The wiggling fingers and the relaxed wrists, that circle the gathering and dredging palms, stimulate all the channels on the hands that connect with the internal organs. The top hand circles inward gathering fresh chi, while the bottom hand circles outward dredging the channels on the hands of bad chi. Wiggling all the fingers, while relaxing the wrists to circle the palms is also good for working all the joints of the fingers and the wrists.

47. TURN BODY, ROTATE THE BALL

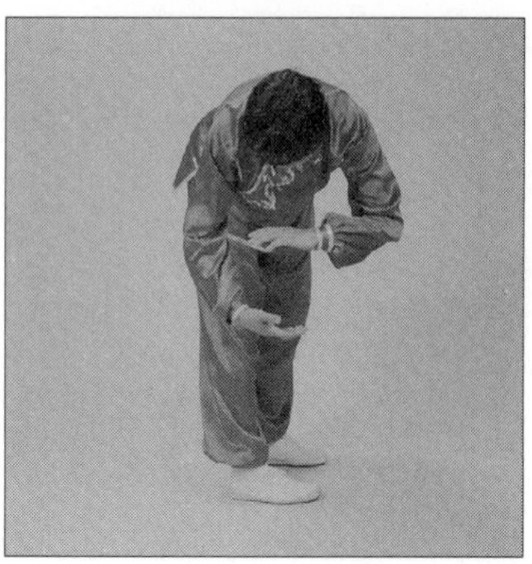

47 a-1. Simultaneously rotate both palms. Bringing the left palm upward, and the right palm downward. The left palm faces the right palm.

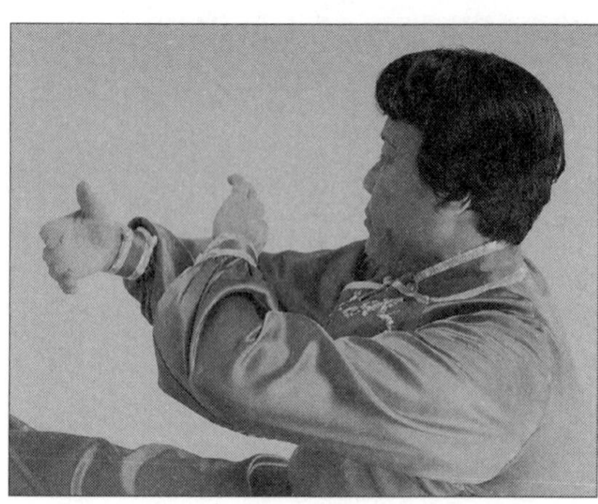

47 a-2. (ANOTHER ANGLE/CLOSE UP) Turn waist gradually back to the left, wiggling the fingers on both hands, while circling the top hand inward (bringing in fresh chi) and circling the bottom hand outward (bringing out bad chi).

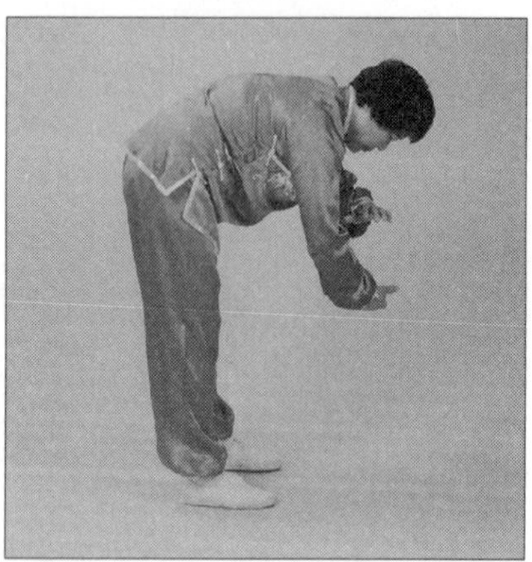

47 b-1. At a slightly faster rate than the previous form, Rotate The Ball, you should have reached the center by the fourth count.

47 b-2. (ANOTHER ANGLE/CLOSE UP) Continue turning the waist gradually to the left, wiggling the fingers on both hands, while circling the top hand inward and circling the bottom hand outward.

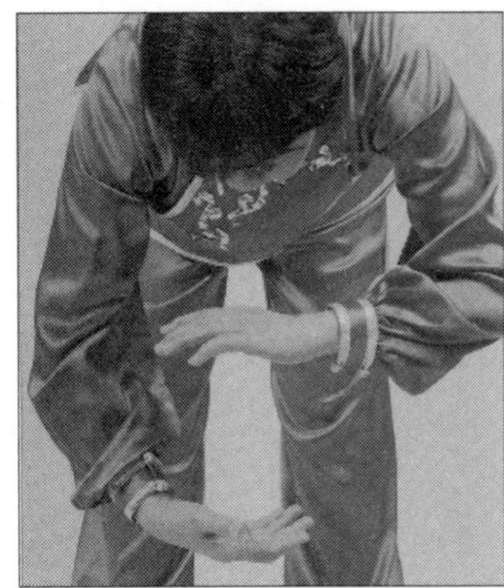

47 c-1. Continue turning all the way to the left. The fingers continue wiggling, while the top circles inward and the bottom hand circles outward.

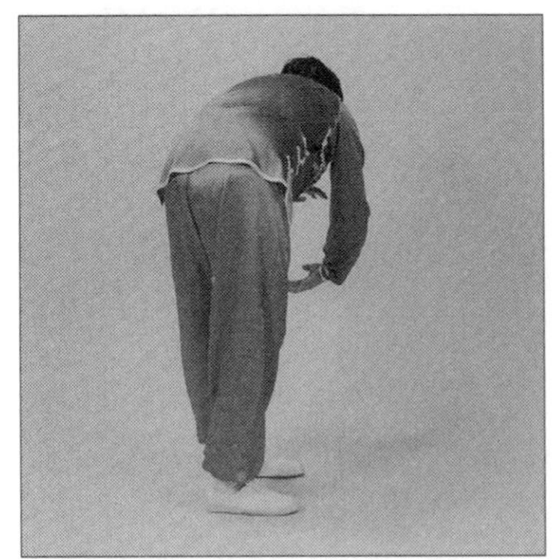

47 c-2. (ANOTHER ANGLE/CLOSE UP) You should reach all the way to the left side by the count of eight. Continue wiggling the fingers, while the top hand continues to circle inward and the bottom hand circles outward. Do not change the palms, while you turn the waist gradually right or back to the center on two more counts.

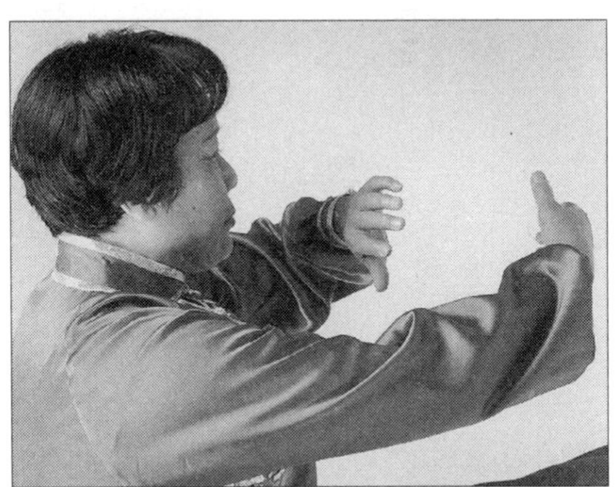

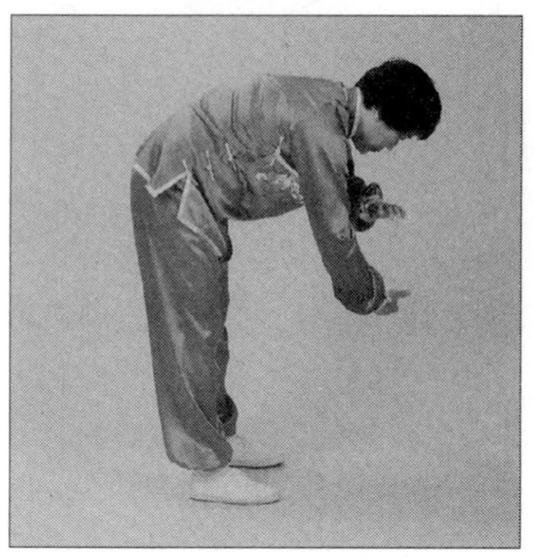

47 d-1. Return to the center from the left side by the tenth count.

CHI ESSENTIALS: See Chi Essentials for Form 46, Rotate The Ball.

48. HOLD AIR

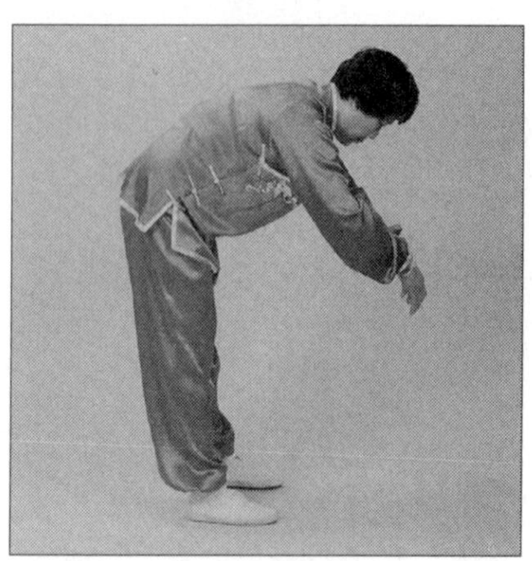

48 a. Let left hand pass down to naturally meet up with the right as you gradually begin to lift torso.

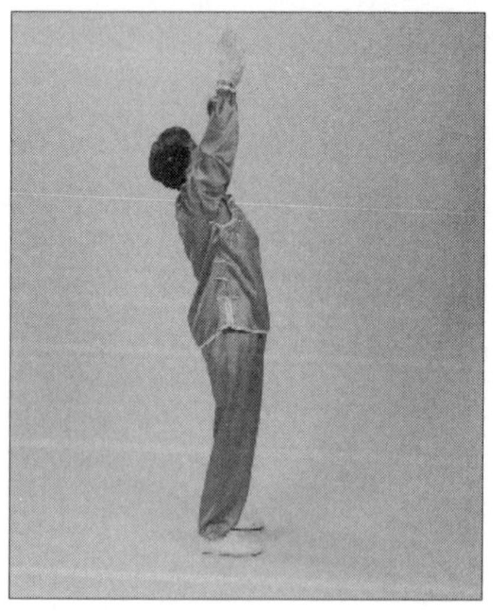

48 b. As the torso comes up, raise the hands upward to the sky. The eyes follow the hands upward. At your fullest extension upwards, turn the palms outward.

48 c. Gradually bend downward at the waist, while letting the palms come outward. As you bend over more, if you can, let the palms gradually turn inward. Between the arms, embrace an imaginary ball. Remember, if you have high blood pressure or heart problems, do not bring the head down past the heart. Keep the legs locked, even if you can't bend over very far. Do not bend the legs, in order to bend over more.

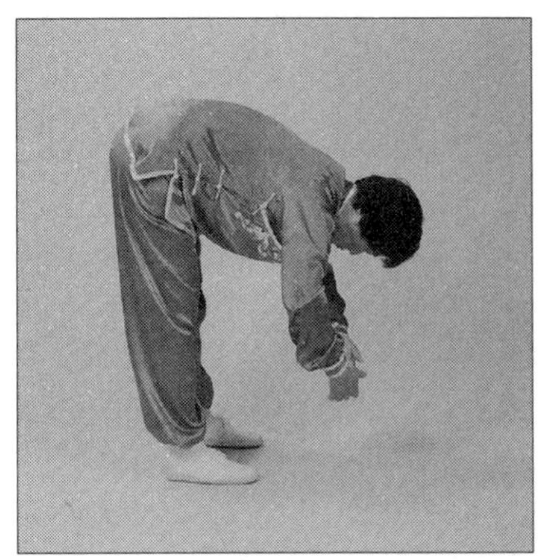

48 d-1. Then without moving the arms, lift the torso straight, bend the knees and sit down as far as possible. However, keep the buttocks tucked, and keep the back as straight as possible; thereby opening the Mingmen point. Keep the knees aligned vertically with the toes. Keep the shoulders and heels down. Pause for a period of time, and focus your energy far into the distance. Relax, and breathe gently. Imagine as if you are sitting on a high chair in front of a tree, and your arms are gently embracing a tree. Don't hold any tightness in the joints. If you can practice embracing a tree in this posture. Notice after a short period of time, how you will not hold any tightness in your joints or limbs, in order to embrace the tree.

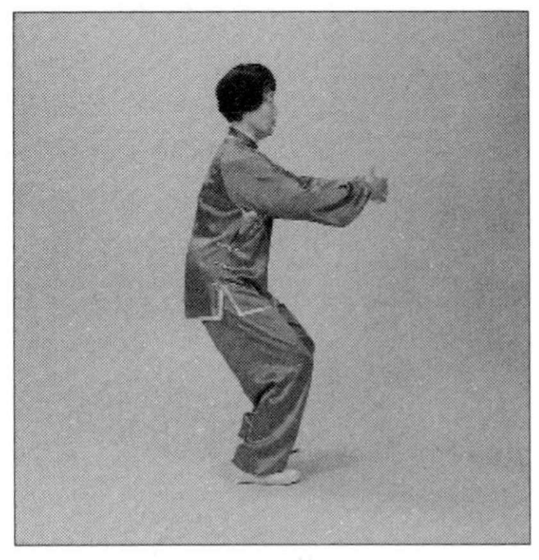

48 d-2. This is an incorrect example of the Hold Air posture. Likely what went wrong is that the arms were raised when coming up; instead of raising the torso, while maintaining the arms in front of the chest to hold up Chi. Furthermore to compensate for tightness being held in the upper limbs, the buttocks protrudes closing the Mingmen ("Life Gate") point. Also the neck is tightened, and out of alignment with the torso. Refer to 48 d-1 for the key points, and a correct visual example.

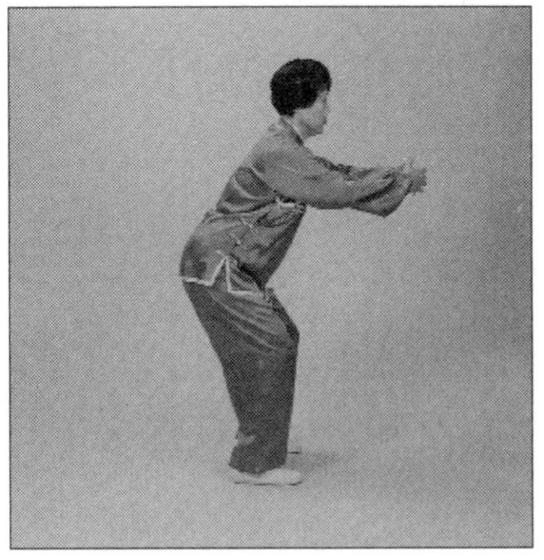

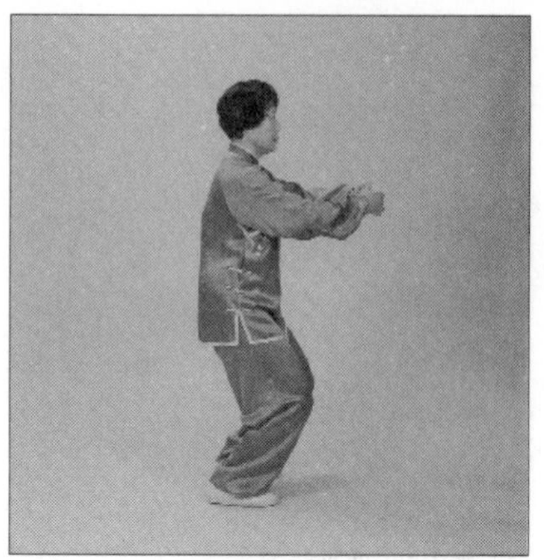

48 d-3. Here is another incorrect example of the Hold Air posture. Here, in order to keep the back straight and to sit deeper, the knees are brought past the vertical alignment with the toes. Remember, it's not important how deep you sit, but how correctly you follow the main points of correct practice. In this way, you will reduce the risk of any injury in your practice. Refer to 48 d-1 for a review of the key points, and a correct visual example.

CHI ESSENTIALS: The movements of the hands upward helps open the three Yin channels on the hands. The movements of the hands downward to hold an imaginary ball helps open the three Yang channels of the hands. When the imaginary ball is held between the arms and without moving the arms you straighten the torso and sit down, the Mingmen point and the Qihu points are opened and stimulated. As you pause and stare into the distance, and sit for a time Chi is collected at the Mingmen point. The Ball shape between the arms may become heavy. This is the Chi building up pressure and developing within your arms' embrace. Try at this time not to hold any tightness whatsoever in your joints, upper limbs, back, or neck. Relax, breathe gently, and let your air and energy inside you circulate on all channels and meridians. Encouraging the Systemic Circulation discussed earlier.

49. PASS THROUGH AIR

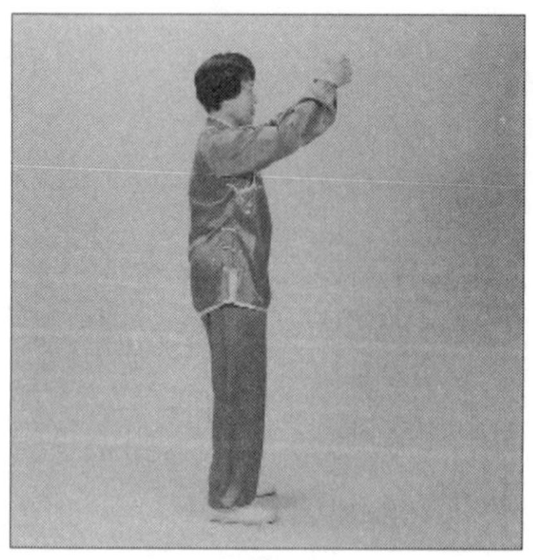

49 a-1. Gradually stand erect from the sitting posture of the previous form, Hold Air, while allowing the hands to gradually come up to the forehead.

49 a-2. (ANOTHER ANGLE/CLOSE UP) The palms face slightly inward, so that the Laogong points on both palms face the Yintang point (located between the eyebrows) and the Upward Dantian. Look straight ahead into the distance.

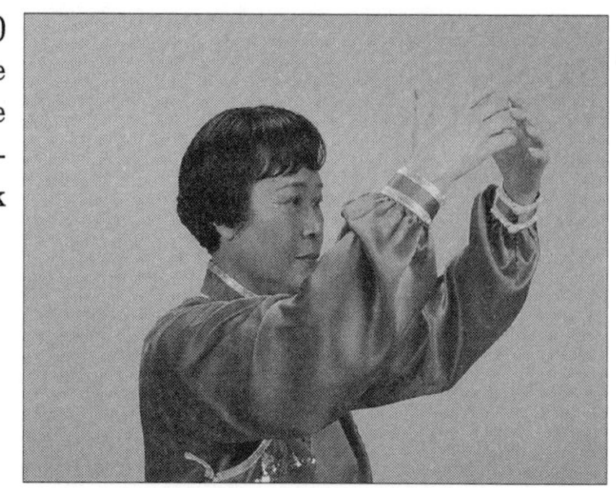

49 b-1. Then gently and gradually allow the arms to descend with the palms still facing inward. Passing through the breast bone. Hold no tightness in the joints or upper limbs. Let your arms come down gently, as if sliding down an imaginary tree trunk that your arms embrace.

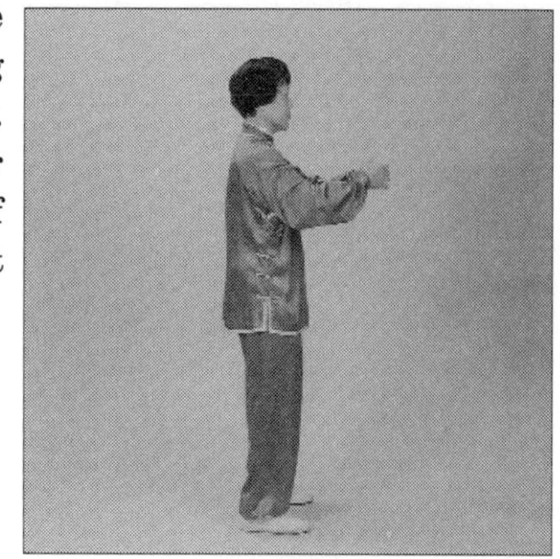

49 b-2. (ANOTHER ANGLE/CLOSE UP) The palms face inward, so that the Laogong points on both palms face the Shanzhong point (located in the center of the breast bone, between the two nipples) and the Middle Dantian. Continue looking far away into the distance.

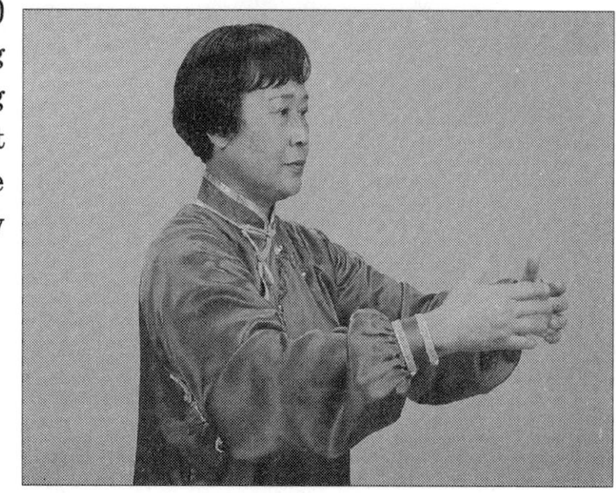

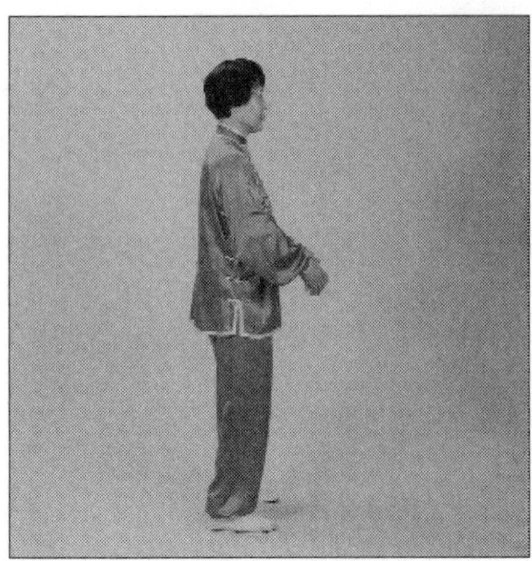

49 c-1. Continue gradually allowing the palms to continue descending to the lower abdomen. Again hold no tightness in the joints or upper limbs.

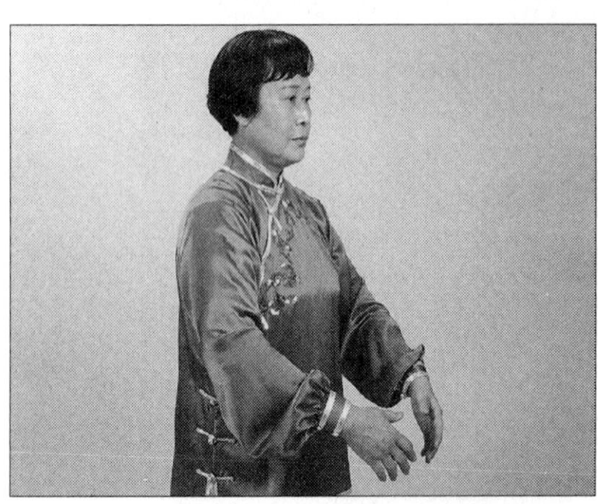

49 c-2. (ANOTHER ANGLE/CLOSE UP) The palms face inward, so that the Laogong points on both palms face the Qihai point (located below the navel, and vertically aligned with the navel) and the Lower Dantian.

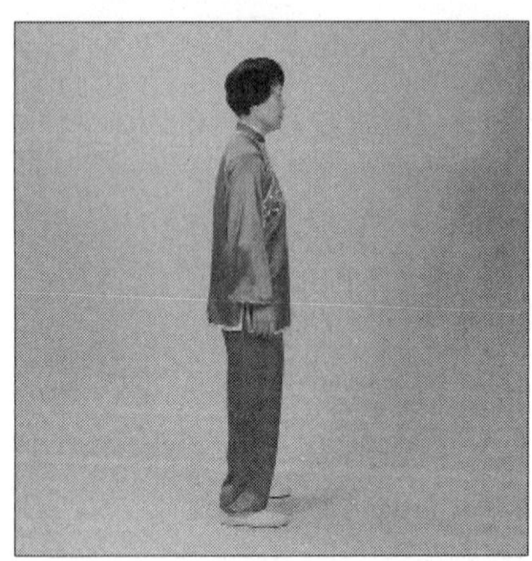

49 d. After a few moments, allow the hands to come all the way down to the sides of the legs. Continue looking straight ahead into the distance. Stand very balanced.

CHI ESSENTIALS: Bring up all the Chi you developed from the previous form, Hold Air. Store this Chi by first pouring it in the Upward Dantian. Then as the hands come down, allow the Chi both externally and internally to come down, to be stored in the Lower Dantian and to continue all the way down through the feet to the Yongquan point (located near the center of the ball of the foot on both feet).

When the Chi reaches the Yongquan point, receive the Earth (Yin) energy to strengthen the body's Yin energy. Also remember, as the hands gently and gradually come down, do not hold any tightness in the joints or upper limbs. Instead, as previously discussed, allow the hands to come down as if sliding down an imaginary tree trunk that your arms embrace.

50. RAISE ARMS

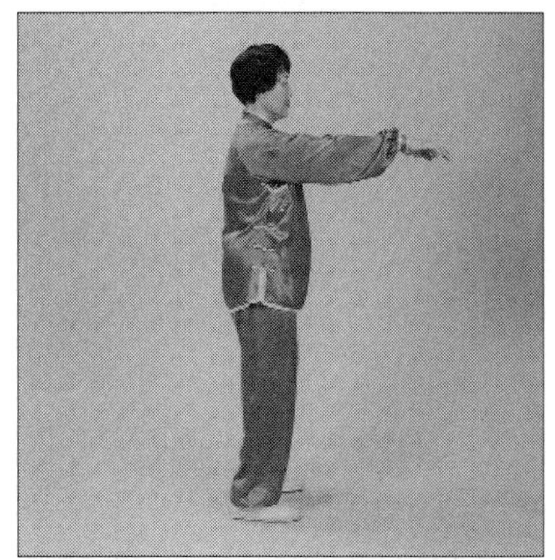

50 a. While gradually moving the weight forward into the balls of the feet (keep the heels on the ground), raise arms to shoulder level. Palms face downward towards the Earth.

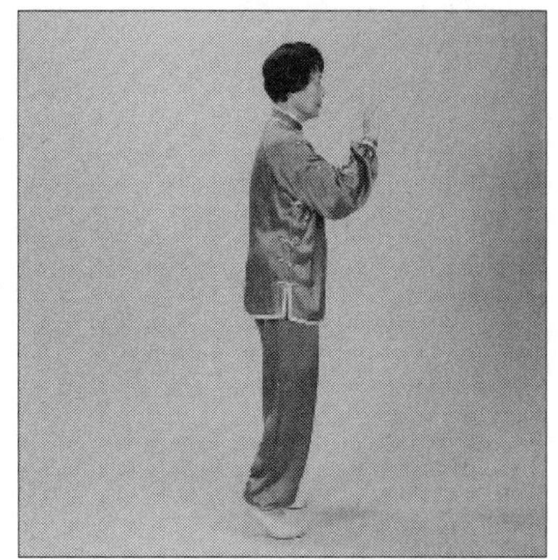

50 b. Then gradually raise the heels, while simultaneously bringing the elbows down. The hands are drawn inward, but remain level with the shoulders. The palms face outward (Yang palms). The heels are raised, preparing for the Heels down method (Force).

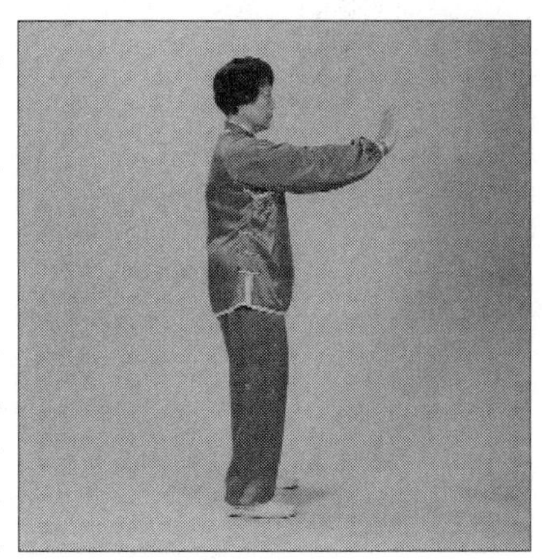

50 c. Then simultaneously thrust the palms forward at shoulder level, while dropping the heels to the ground solidly with the body's weight (Heels down method with force.).

Continue looking straight ahead.

CHI ESSENTIALS: When the hands raise up to shoulder level, the Yin channels on both hands are stimulated. When the elbows gradually drop and the hands are drawn in the Laogong point in the center of the palm on both hands are stimulated and opened. Simultaneously while the heels are gradually raised the Yongquan points on both feet are stimulated and opened.

When the heels drop suddenly with the body's weight striking the ground firmly, this shocks the system. Sending the Yin energy upward, and the Yang energy downward suddenly for the purpose of dredging the channels of bad chi. Because the hands push out with as much force as the dropping heels, the bad chi is also dispelled out from the hands, as well as the feet. Because both upper and lower limbs are meant to act simultaneously, Yin and Yang balance in the system is the ultimate result once bad chi is sent out.

51. DROP WINGS

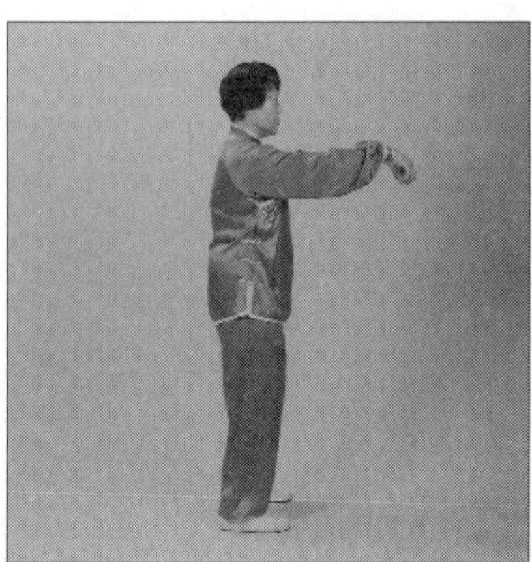

51-1. While maintaining the arms at shoulder level let the fingers on both hands drop to form Eagle's Beak with hands. Continue looking straight ahead.

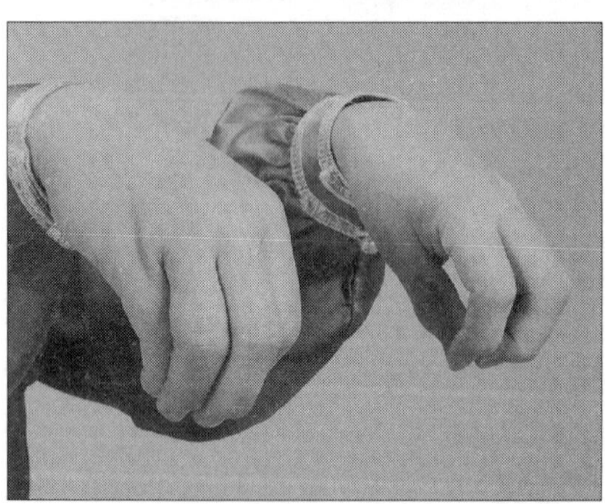

51-2. (ANOTHER ANGLE/CLOSE UP) While forming Eagle's Beaks with the hands, do not hold any tightness in the elbows or shoulders. The fingers and wrists should not be limp, nor should they be tightened to form the Eagle's Beaks.

CHI ESSENTIALS: The five fingers come together and point downward to dispel bad chi.

52. FLAP WINGS TO THE BACK

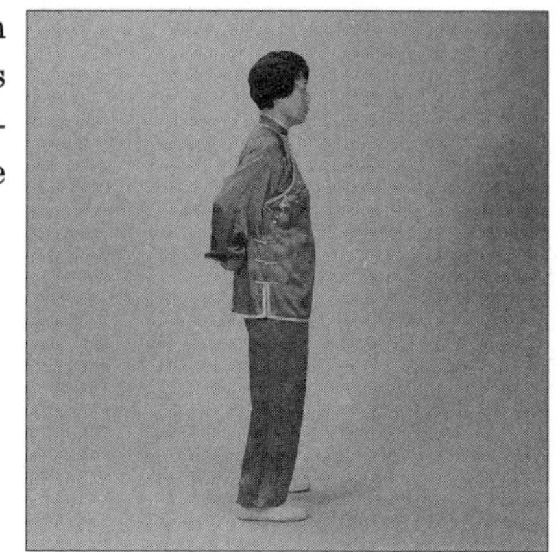

52-1. Without increasing any tightness in your shoulders, elbows, joints, or limbs bring, the Eagle's Beaks gradually downward and behind the body to the small of the back.

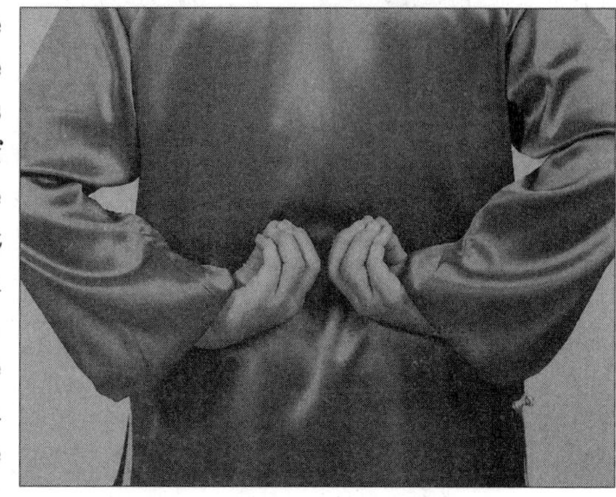

52-2. (ANOTHER ANGLE/CLOSE UP) The Eagle's Beaks are placed in the small of the back, so that the Hegu points on both hands contact the Shenshu points on both sides of the Mingmen point (located opposite the navel on the back). The fingers point upward, with the thumbs and forefingers on both hands resting on the small of the back.

*Once the Eagle's Beaks reach the small of the back, relax a moment, then inhale gently and deeply into the diaphragm. Exhale gently and gradually. When you reach near the end of your exhale, vibrate the Eagle's Beaks on both hands firmly in the small of the back. Repeat this two more times for a total of three repetitions.

CHI ESSENTIALS: As you gradually bring the Eagle's Beaks back behind the body, gather fresh chi on the Hegu points on both hands, and place the fresh Chi in the Shenshu points located on both sides of the Mingmen (life Gate) point. This places fresh Chi in the Kidneys, and stimulates both the Small Intestine and Urinary Bladder Channels. The vibrating of the Eagle's Beaks at these points helps to strengthen the Kidney to overcome or ward off kidney problems or dysfunction, back problems, and impotence.

53. FLY UP TO ONE SIDE

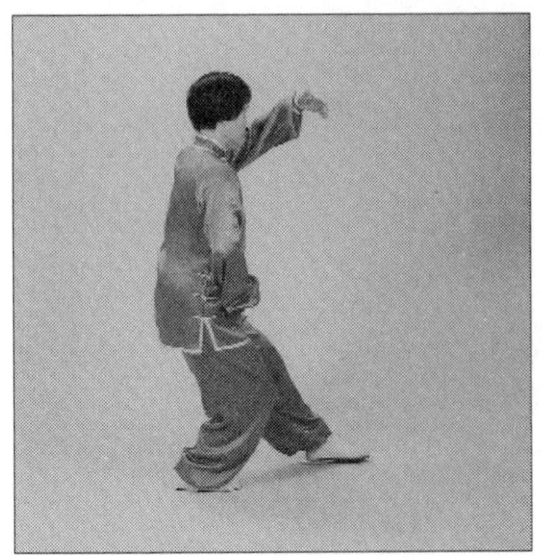

53 a-1. Change the Eagle's Beaks, used in the previous form, to open palms. Turn the waist right, while bringing the hands down past the hips and forward. Turn the waist gradually left, sink the weight into the right leg, and gently extend the left foot forward forming an Empty stance (Outer Edge of the Foot). Simultaneously, bring the left palm up to face the forehead, and bring the right hand inward to face the lower abdomen. Look at the left palm.

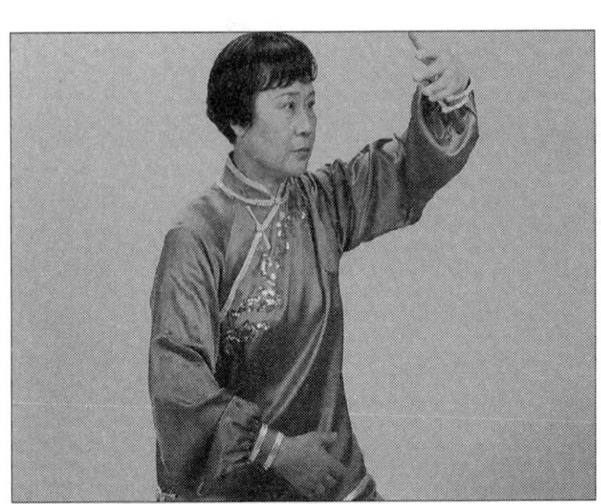

53 a-2. (ANOTHER ANGLE/CLOSE UP) The fingers on the upper hand point to the right and slightly downward. The fingers on the lower hand point to the left and slightly downward. The Laogong point on the left palm faces inward toward the Yintang point (located between the eyebrows) and the Upward Dantian, while the right palm faces inward towards the Lower Dantian. Turn the waist 45-60 degrees left from the center line.

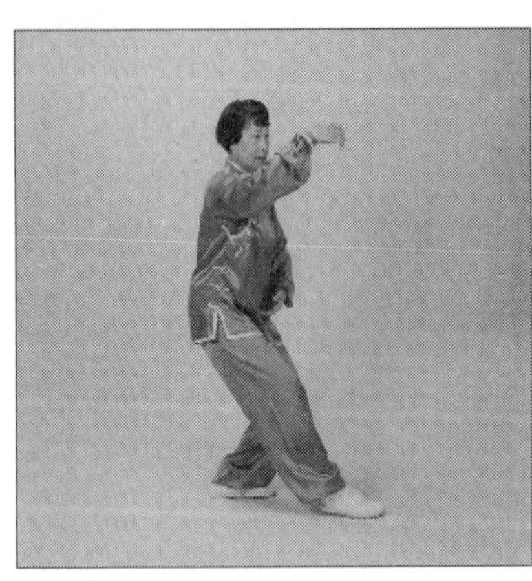

53 b. Turn the waist a little more left to begin changing the palms. Gradually bringing the left palm down to face inward towards the Lower Dantian, and gradually bringing the right palm up to face inward to the Yintang point and the Upward Dantian. Sink the weight into the left leg, and gently extend the right foot forward forming an Empty stance (Outer Edge of the Foot). Turn the waist right 45-60 degrees right from the center line to complete the palm change. Look at the right palm.

*Repeat movements 53 a-1 and 53 b four more times; taking four more steps forward for a total of six forward steps, then do movement 53 c.

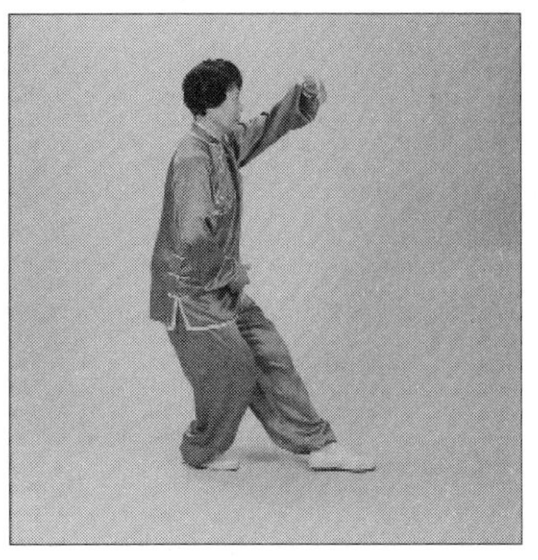

53 c. Similar to movement 53 a-1, however, take a seventh step forward crossing the left foot over the right foot's channel. Do not turn the torso to the left. Rather stay on the center line to contact the next form, Turn Body.

**There are a total of seven steps in this form. Performed as left, right, left, right, left, right, and left. However, the last step is different then the first six steps. Utilizing a cross over step as described and shown in movement 53 c.

CHI ESSENTIALS: This form stimulates the Yang channels on both hands. The upward hand contacts the Upward Dantian each time, while the lower hand contacts the Lower Dantian. The step forward each time forming the Empty stance (Outer Edge of the Foot) opens the Yongquan point, and the Earth's energy is contacted and absorbed. The twisting of the waist in this form helps adjust the spinal nerve and stimulate the Dazhui ("Big Vertebra") point located on the neck bone.

54. TURN BODY

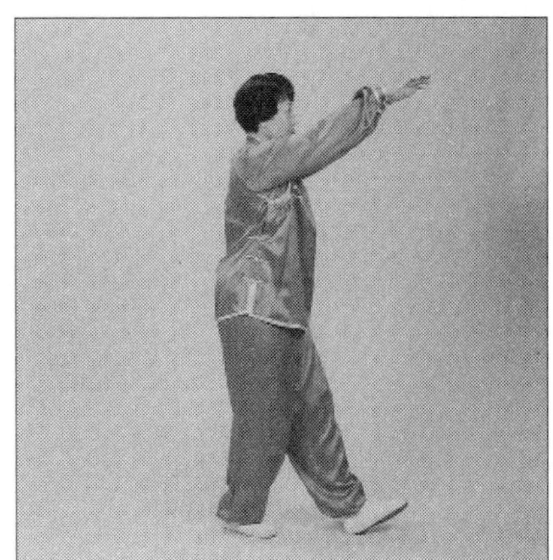

54 a. Sit back in the right leg, while simultaneously raising the left toe, and raising the arms and Shaking Palms upward. Eyes follow the hands.

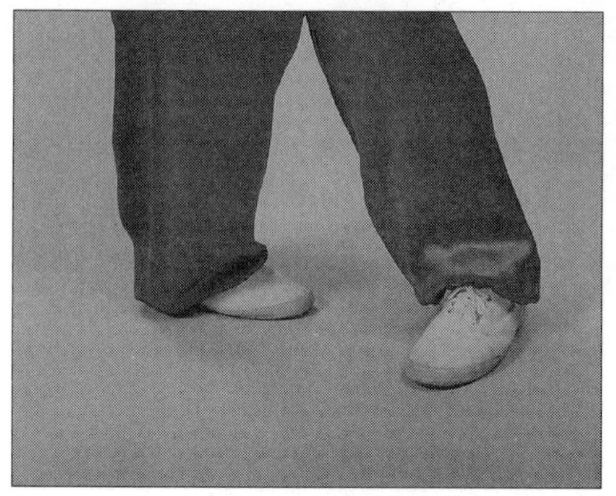

54 b. (ANOTHER ANGLE/CLOSE UP) Next, pivot on the left heel, and turn the left toe right as far as possible. Then move the weight into the left leg. Pivoting on the right heel, turn the right toe 180 degrees right. The arms continuing quivering the Shaking Palms upward, as the body assumes a new direction.

CHI ESSENTIALS: For this transitional movement, the turning of the body with the weight emphasized in the heels opens the Stomach Channel. The turning of the waist works the Dai Meridian.

55. FLY UP TO THE SKY

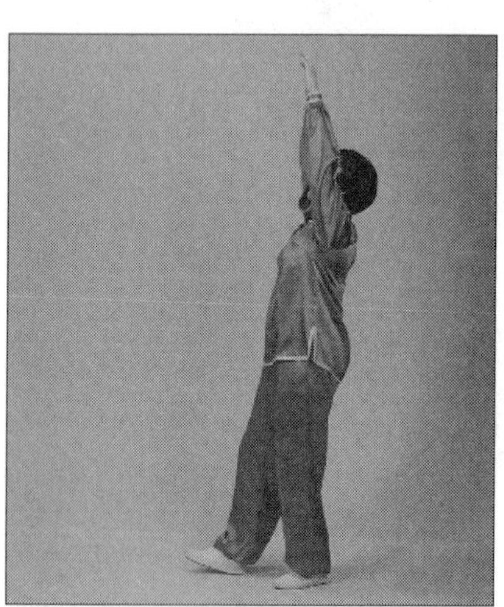

55 a. The Shaking Palms continue upward to the sky, as the body assumes a new direction 180 degrees with the previous. The weight is mostly in the left leg with the right toe raised up. Eyes continue following the hands.

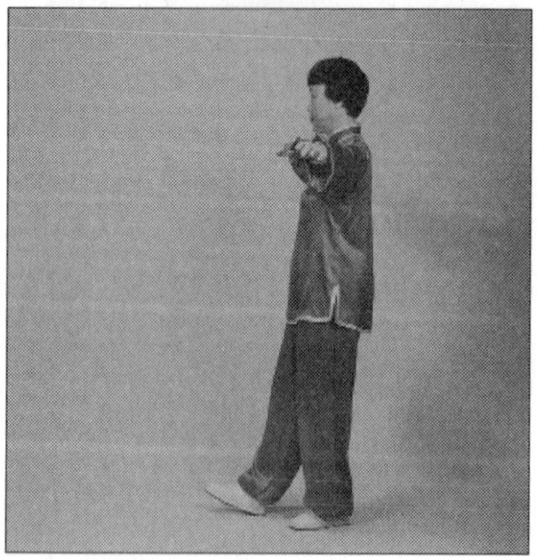

55 b. With the weight still predominately in the left leg and the right toe raised, lower the quivering arms and Shaking Palms downward and outward to shoulder level. The Shaking Palms face downward.

CHI ESSENTIALS: When the Shaking Palms come down the 3 Yin channels on the arms and hands are stimulated.

56. SKIM OVER WATER

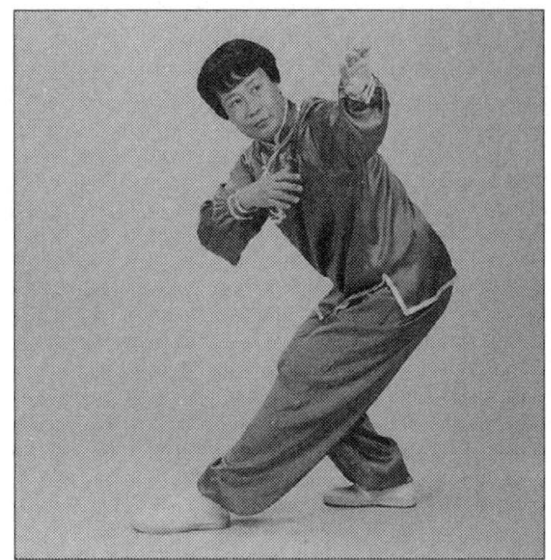

56 a. Bring the shaking arms right first, while moving the weight forward into the right leg (Transition). The right arm is extended away from the body to the right at shoulder level, while the left palm comes in and faces the right Qihu point.

Then gradually sink the weight into the right leg, and gently extend the left foot forward forming an Empty stance (Ball of the Foot). Bend the torso forward, bring the Shaking Palms left to pass over the tops of the legs, and gradually bring the continuous Shaking Palms to the left side of the body. The left Shaking Palm is extended out at shoulder level, and now faces outward from the body. The right Shaking Palm faces inward to the left Qihu.

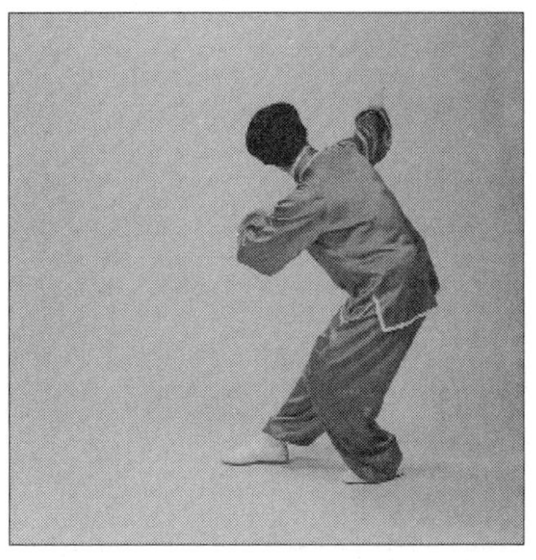

56 b. Then stand gradually stand erect, move the weight forward into the left leg. Then gradually sink the weight into the left leg, and gently extend the right leg forward forming an Empty stance (Ball of the Foot). Bend the torso forward, bring the Shaking Palms right to pass over the tops of the legs, and gradually bring the continuous Shaking Palms to the right side of the body. The right Shaking Palm is extended out at shoulder level, and now faces outward from the body. The left Shaking Palm faces inward to the right Qihu.

*Repeat movements 56 a and 56 b four more times; taking four more steps forward for a total of six steps, then do movement 56 c.

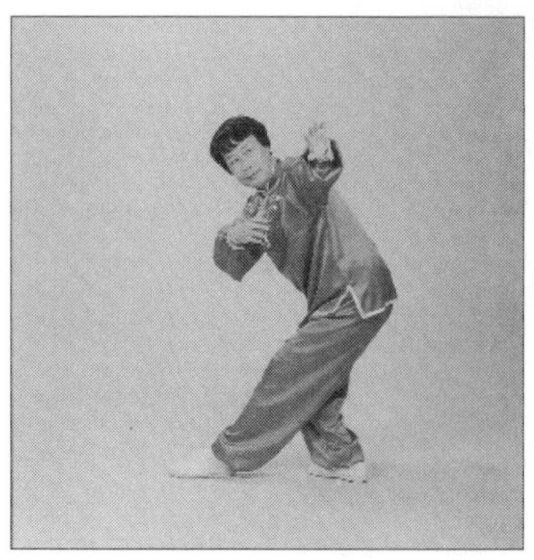

56 c. Similar to movement 56 a, however, take a seventh step forward crossing the left over the right foot's channel. The shaking arms complete a full repetition more by coming to the left side.

**There are a total of seven steps in this form. Performed as left, right, left, right, left, right, and left. However, the last step is different then the first six steps. Utilizing a cross over step as described and shown in movement 56 c.

CHI ESSENTIALS: The form, Skim Over Water, stimulates all 12 Channels, exercises the spine (especially the lower back), and opens and works the Dai Meridian. The Shaking Palms help speed up the flow of Chi and blood. The kidneys are strengthened because of the up and down movement, combined with the turning of the waist.

57. TURN BODY

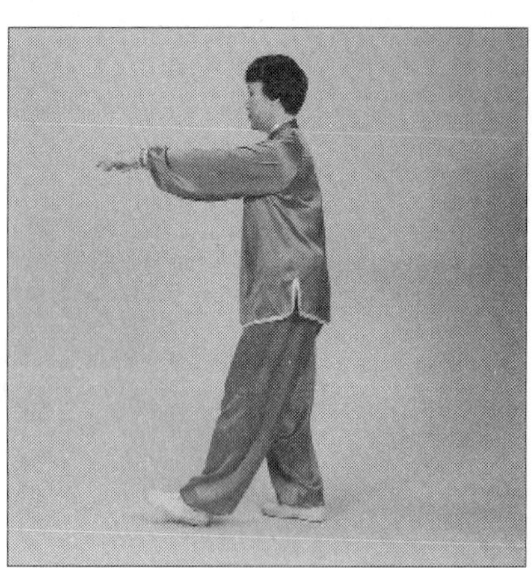

57 a. After the previous form, Skim Over Water, bring the left and the right Shaking Palms to the center in front of the lower abdomen. Move the weight back into the right leg, extend the Shaking Palms forward, and raise the left toe upward.

57 b. Pivot on the left heel, turn the left toe inward and to your right as far as possible. Continuing turning and raising the Shaking Palms upward, and gradually move the weight back into the left leg. The right toe raises, as you pivot on the right heel 180 degrees, and begin turning backwards to the right. The eyes follow the hands.

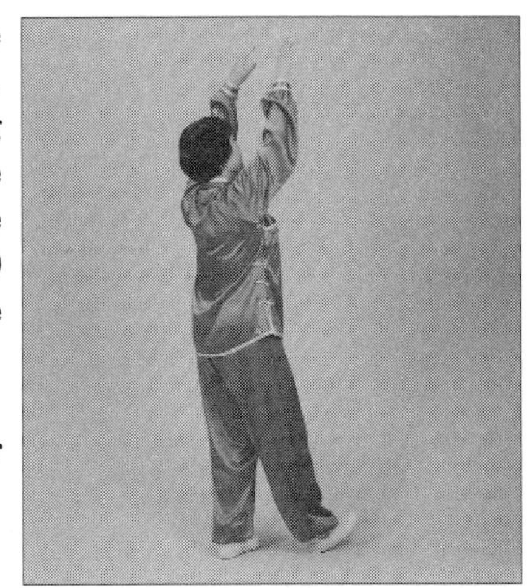

CHI ESSENTIALS: See Chi Essentials for form 54, Turn Body.

58. FLY UPWARD

58 a. Continue shaking the palms upward. The toes on the right foot point 135 degrees right and away from the previous direction. The right toe is still raised, weight in the left leg, as the palms turn outward.

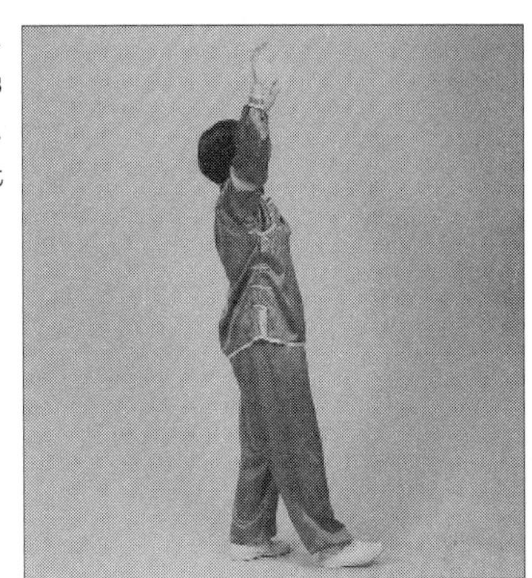

58 b. Bring the Shaking Palms downward to the shoulder level, while gradually moving the weight forward into the right foot (the right toe points 45 degrees to the right). Simultaneously, gradually raise the left heel off the ground. When the Shaking Palms reach the shoulder level, stop shaking the palms.

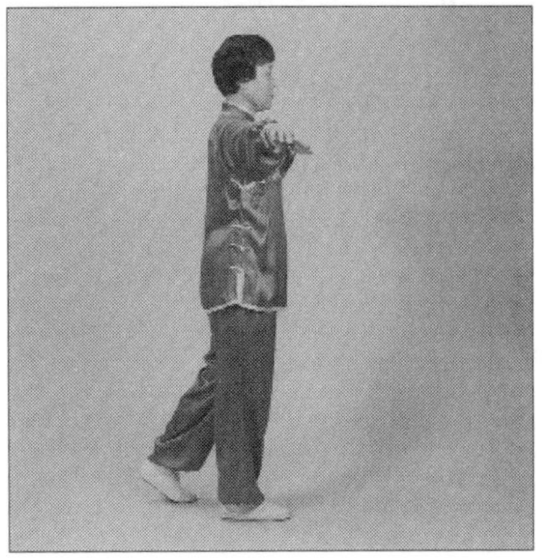

CHI ESSENTIALS: See Chi Essentials for Form 55, Fly Up To The Sky.

59. LOOK FOR FOOD

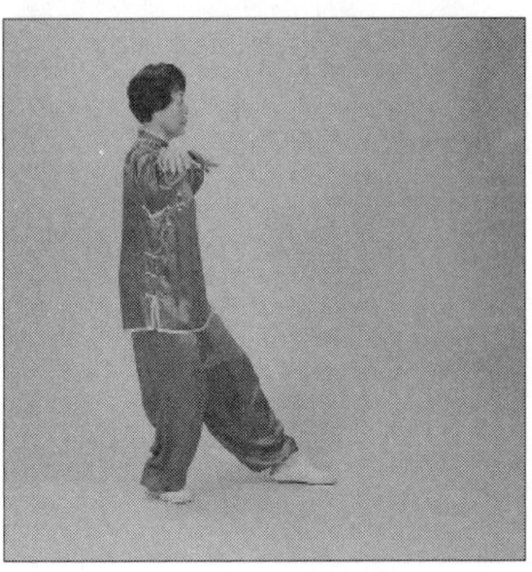

59 a. Sink the weight into the right leg, and gently extend the left foot forward forming an Empty stance (Ball of the Foot). The eyes look straight ahead,

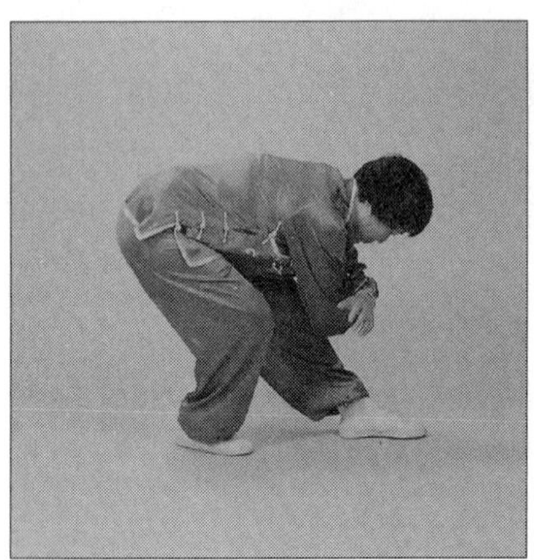

59 b-1. Then bend the body forward and over at the torso, while simultaneously bringing the arms down to cross each other with the left arm on top.

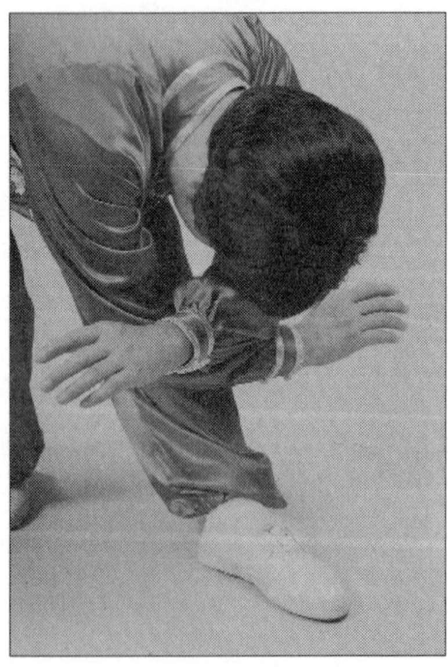

59 b-2. (ANOTHER ANGLE/CLOSE UP) The head relaxes over and maintains the same line with the torso. The arms don't merely swing down, cross, and separate without being connected with the up and down movement of the torso. Remember when the body goes down it acts as a spring that contracts, and the arms, relaxed, follow the torso's movements downward. When the body comes up the arms uncross and gently come up and out to shoulder level.

59 c. The torso relaxes and gradually comes up from the previous movement, while simultaneously the arms gradually come up, separate, and gradually extend out at shoulder level. Then turn the left heel inward, so the toes on the left foot point 45 degrees to the left.

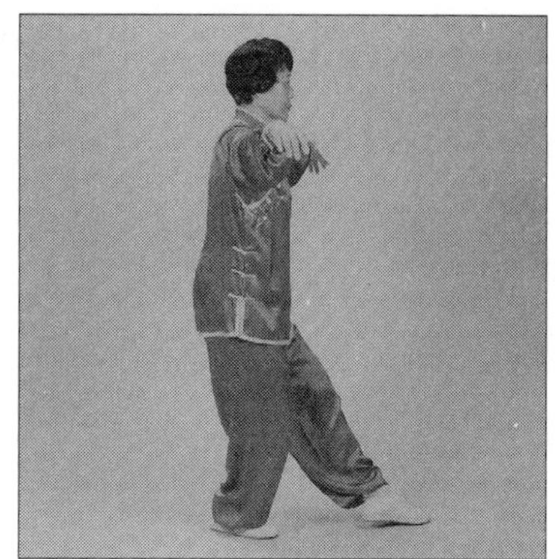

59 d. Move the weight forward onto the left leg, and gently extend the right leg forward forming a right Empty stance (Ball of the Foot). Gradually sink the weight into the left leg, bend forward and over at the torso, and bring the arms down to cross each other with the right arm on top.

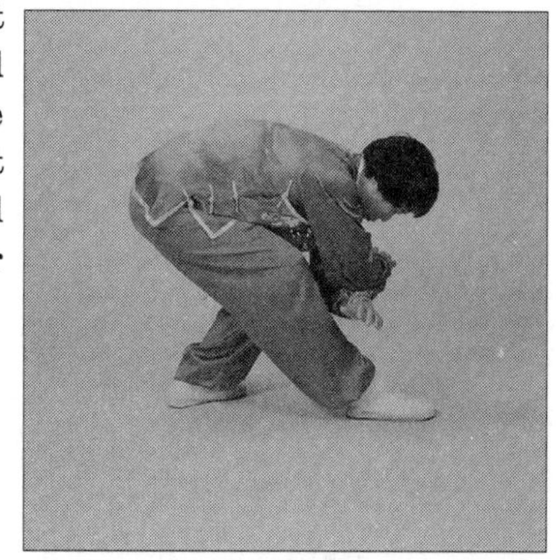

59 e. The torso relaxes and gradually comes up from the previous movement, while simultaneously the arms gradually come up, separate, and gradually extend out at shoulder level. Then turn the right heel inward, so the toes on the left foot point 45 degrees to the right.

*Repeat movements 59 a, 59 b-1, 59 c, 59, d, and 59 e four more times; taking four more steps forward for a total of six steps, then do movement 59 f.

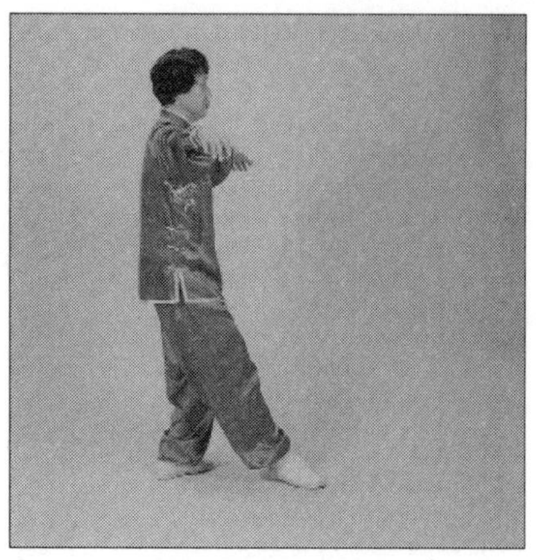

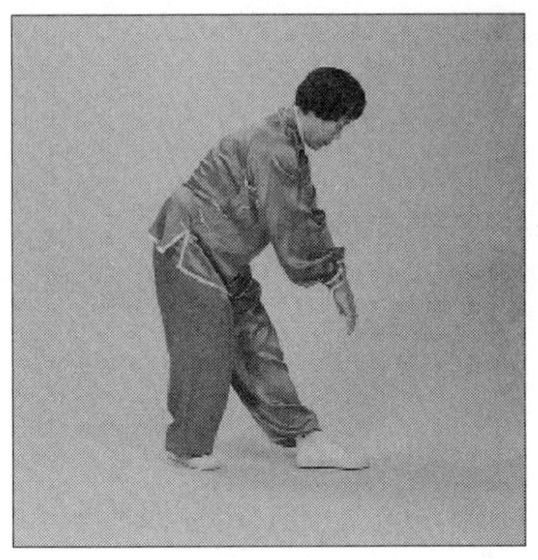

59 f. Similar to movement 59 a, however, take a seventh step forward crossing the left foot over the right foot's channel. Also do not let the arms come up to shoulder level, as the torso comes up. Instead the hands come up towards the lower abdomen, and the next form, 60. , Turn Body, is contacted.

**There are a total of seven steps in this form. Performed as left, right, left, right, left, right, and left. However, the last step is different then the first six steps. Utilizing a cross over step as described and shown in movement 59 f.

CHI ESSENTIALS: The movement in this form opens the 12 channels on the feet and hands. Also the movement of this form, if done correctly, will train the body to perform the Pulmonary Circulation (The joining of Du and Ren Meridians, and small orbit of chi circulation.). When the torso comes up the Chi will naturally come up the Du Meridian, when the torso goes down the Chi will naturally fall down the Ren Meridian like a waterfall.

That's why it's important to let the body be like a spring contracting downward, and bouncing in the back of the waist, before the hands uncross and the torso comes upward. The arms shouldn't swing without being connected to the bouncing or spring like quality assumed by the torso. Otherwise if the arms just swing, the torso is on it's own to move up and down, and the natural force of momentum will be unable to employ the limbs holistically. The arms, when joined with the torso, can help the torso to gather momentum to go up and down. Then the Chi can be free to flow on the Du and Ren Meridians as indicated, and the Pulmonary Circulation more effectively trained and accomplished.

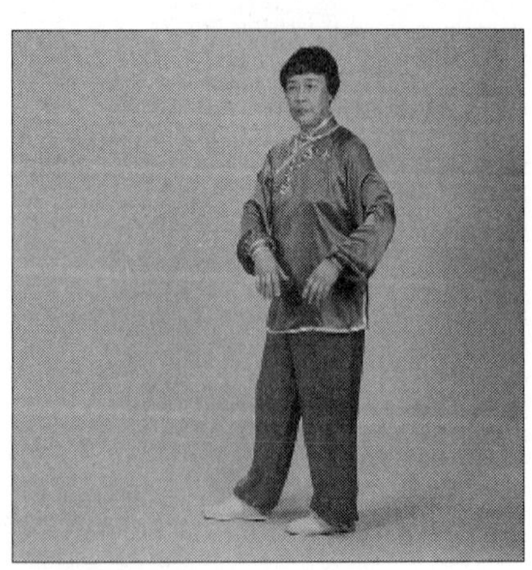

60. TURN BODY

60. Straighten up the body, bring the palms inward to face the lower abdomen, and pivot on the heels 180 degrees to the right. The toes on the right foot point 135 degrees right from the previous direction. The hands remain in front of the lower abdomen, palms facing inward.

CHI ESSENTIALS: As the body comes up, the Chi comes up the Du Meridian (as in the previous form). After finishing it's route on the Du Meridian, instead of continuing the circulation down the Ren Meridian, bring the Chi down to the Lower Dantian to be stored. Remain stable while turning. As the hands stay down in front of the lower abdomen, encouraging the storage of Chi in the Lower Dantian.

61. LOOK FOR THE NEST

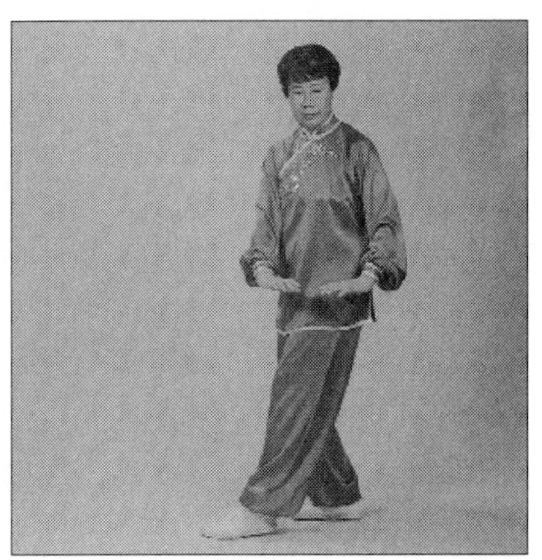

61 a-1. (LEFT) With the toes on the right foot pointing straight ahead, shift the weight into the right foot, and gently extend the left foot straight forward forming the left Empty stance (Ball of the Foot). The torso faces left. The palms change to Pressing palms, and push downward from the abdomen to the side of the left hip. The wrists gradually flex and the palms push downward, as the fingers on both hands point towards each other. Keep the space between the thumb and forefinger open. The eyes look at the hands.

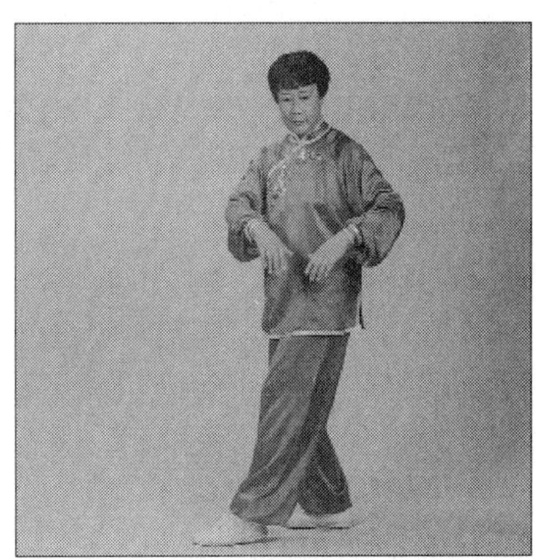

61 a-2. Gradually relax the hands, wrists, and elbows and let them come up slightly. Don't let the hands rise above the breast bone level. Continue watching the hands.

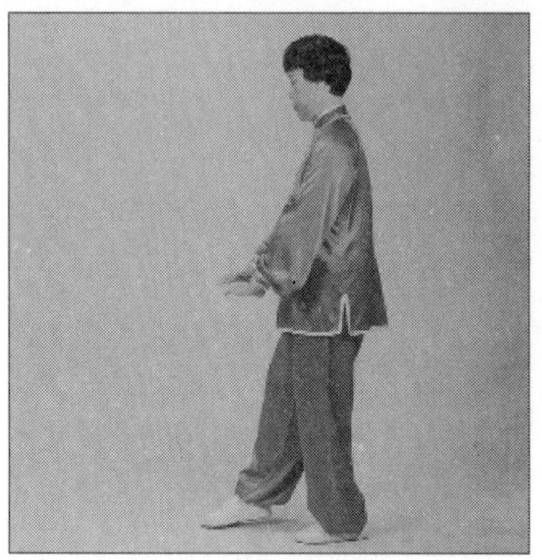

61 b-1. (MIDDLE) With the toes on both feet pointing straight ahead, gradually turn the torso right to face in the same direction as the toes on both feet. Move the weight forward into the left foot, and gently extend the right foot straight forward forming the right Empty stance (Ball of the Foot). Press the palms downward to the lower abdomen. The wrists gradually flex and the palms push downward, as the fingers on both hands point towards each other. Keep the space between the thumb and forefinger open. The eyes look at the hands.

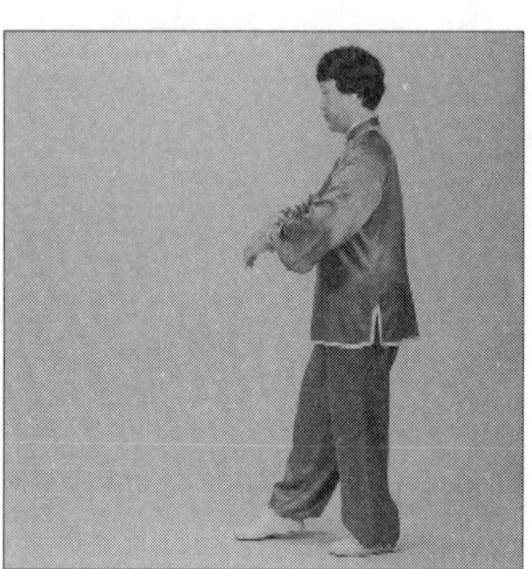

61 b-2. Gradually relax the hands, wrists, and elbows and let them come up slightly. Don't let the hands rise above the breast bone level. Continue watching the hands.

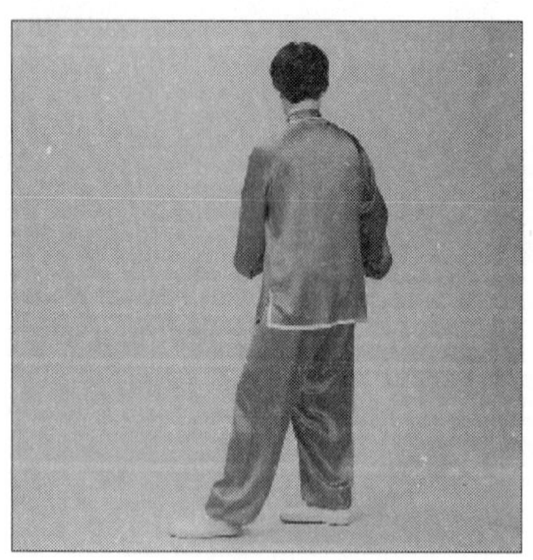

61 c-1. (RIGHT/WITH LEFT FOOT FORWARD) With the toes on both feet pointing straight ahead, turn the torso more to the right. Move the weight forward into the right foot, and gently extend the left foot straight forward forming the left Empty stance (Ball of the Foot). Press the palms downward to the side of the right hip. the palms face downward towards the Earth, the wrists gradually flex, and the fingers on both hands point towards each other. Keep the space between the thumb and forefinger open. The eyes look at the hands.

61 c-2. Gradually relax the hands, wrists, and elbows and let them come up slightly. Don't let the hands rise above the breast bone level. Continue watching the hands.

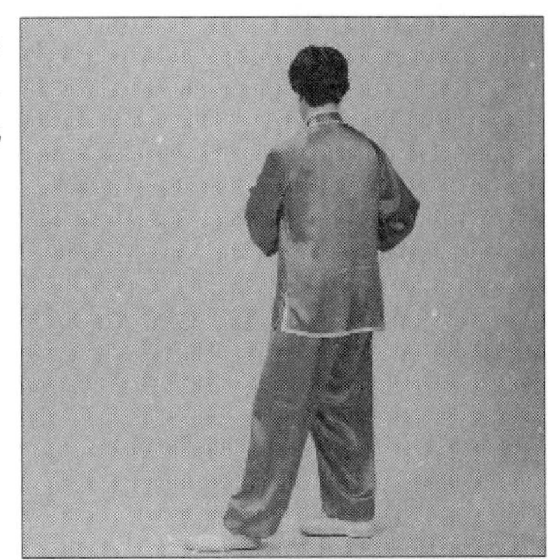

61 d-1. (RIGHT/WITH RIGHT FOOT FORWARD) With the toes on both feet pointing forward, and maintain the torso facing the right side. Move the weight forward into the left foot, and gently extend the right foot straight forward forming the right Empty stance (Ball of the Foot). Press the palms downward to the right side of the hip. The palms face downward towards the Earth, the wrists gradually flex, and the fingers on both hands point towards each other. Keep the space between the thumb and forefinger open. The eyes look at the hands.

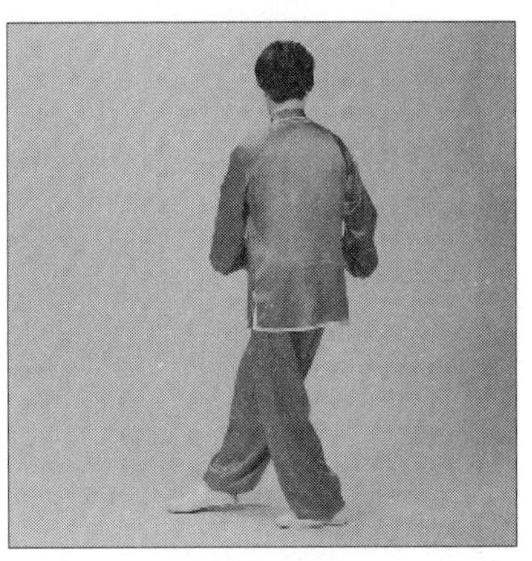

61 d-2. Gradually relax the hands, wrists, and elbows and let them come up slightly. Don't let the hands rise above the breast bone level. Continue watching the hands.

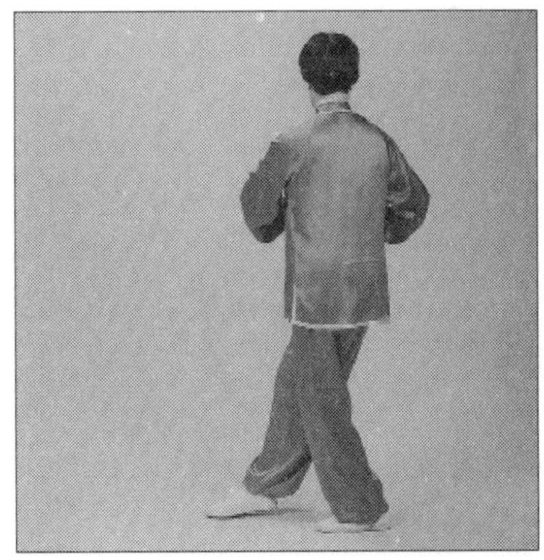

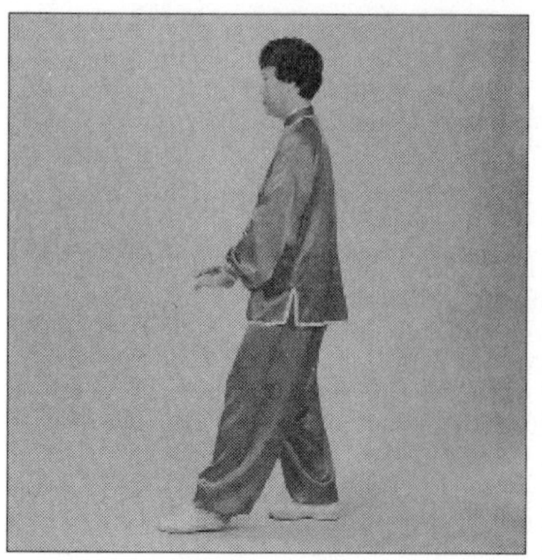

61 e-1. (MIDDLE) With the toes on both feet pointing forward, turn the torso left to face in the same direction as the toes on both feet. Move the weight forward into the right foot, and gently extend the left foot straight forward forming the left Empty stance (Ball of the Foot). Press the palms, and push the palms downward to the lower abdomen. The wrists gradually flex and the palms push downward, as the fingers on both hands point towards each other. Keep the space between the thumb and forefinger open. The eyes look at the hands.

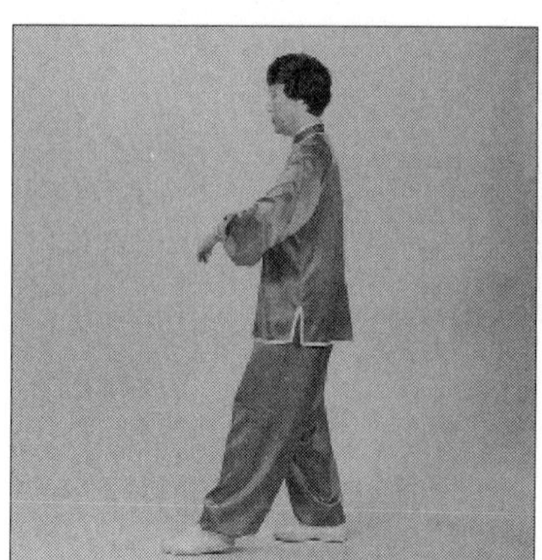

61 e-2. Gradually relax the hands, wrists, and elbows and let them come up slightly. Don't let the hands rise above the breast bone level. Continue watching the hands.

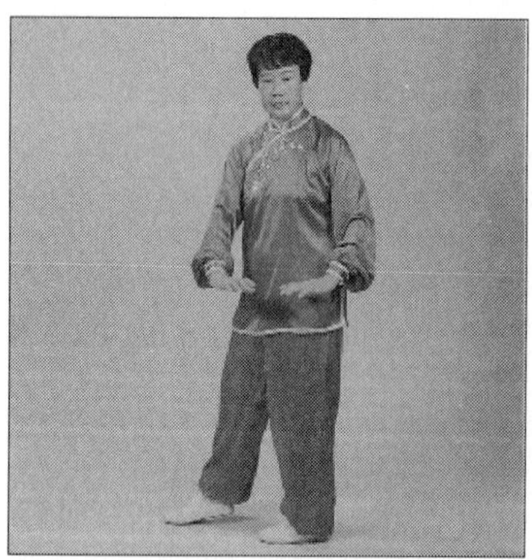

61 f-1. (LEFT) With the toes on both feet pointing forward, turn the torso more left. Move the weight forward into the left foot, and gently extend the right foot forward forming the right Empty stance (Ball of the Foot). Press the palms, and push the palms downward to the left side of the hip. The wrists gradually flex and the palms push downward, as the fingers on both hands point towards each other. Keep the space between the thumb and forefinger open. The eyes look at the hands.

61 f-2. Gradually relax the hands, wrists, and elbows and let them come up slightly. Don't let the hands rise above the breast bone level. Continue watching the hands.

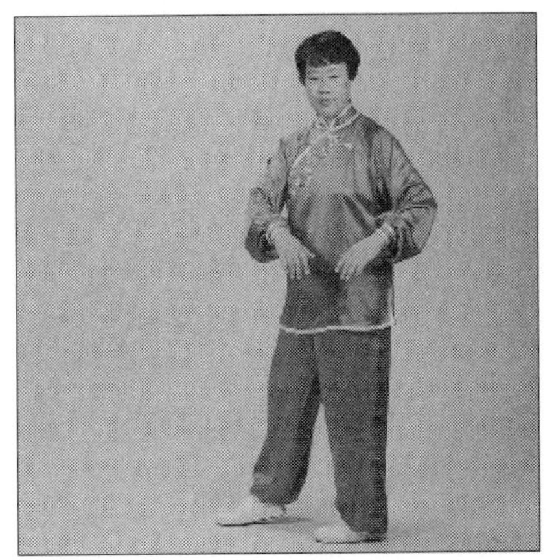

61 g-1. (MIDDLE) With the toes on both feet pointing forward, turn the torso right to face in the same direction as the toes on both feet. Move the weight forward into the right foot, and gently extend the left foot straight forward forming the left Empty stance (Ball of the Foot). Press the palms, and push the palms downward to the lower abdomen. The wrists gradually flex and the palms push downward, as the fingers on both hands point towards each other. Keep the space between the thumb and forefinger opened. The eyes look at the palms.

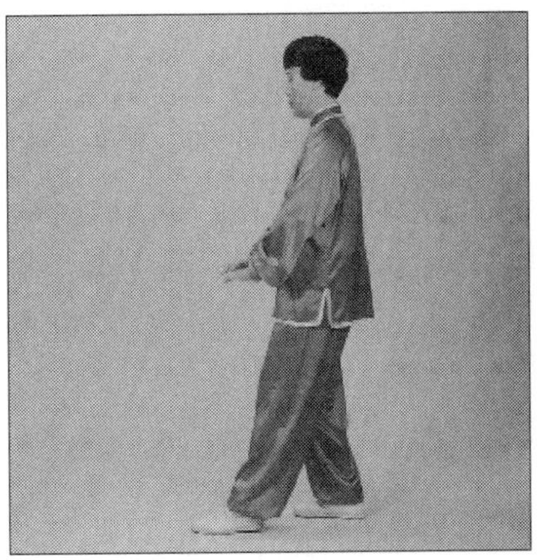

CHI ESSENTIALS: Pressing the palms downward encourages the Triple Warmer Channel to dispel bad chi. When the palms relax, the palms shouldn't come up higher than the Middle Dantian level.

62. TURN BODY AND SWIM

62 a. Raise the left toe, and begin shaking the arms and palms outward and upward.

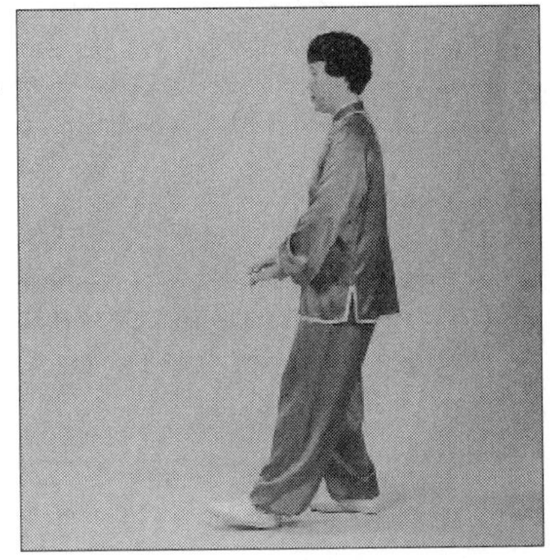

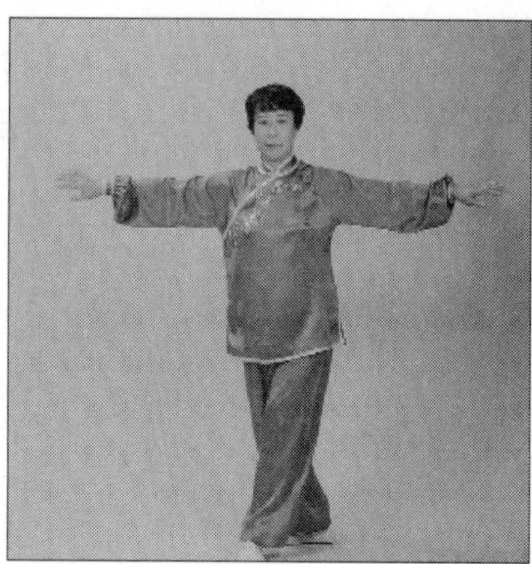

62 b. The palms continue shaking, as the arms spread outward to shoulder level. The left foot pivots 90 degrees to the left. The torso turns back to face the original direction. The eyes look forward.

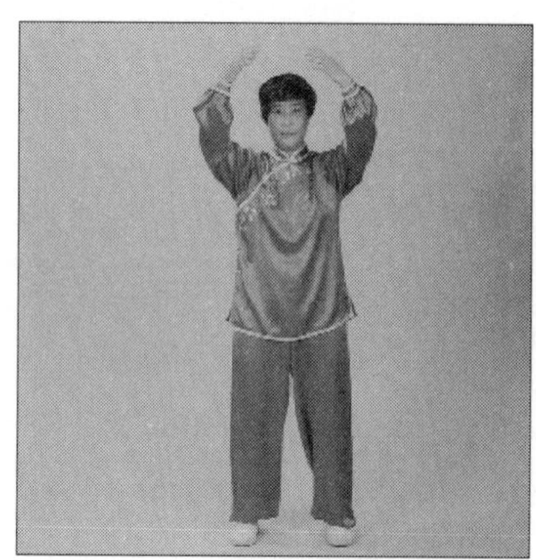

62 c. The palms continue shaking, and the arms move upward to above the forehead level. While simultaneously, the right foot steps up parallel with the left. The palms face downward and slightly inward. The elbows point slightly outward and downward. The eyes look forward.

CHI ESSENTIALS: This form encourages stimulation on the Upward, Middle, and Lower Dantians. Also the form helps open, cleanse, and heighten the senses associated with the seven apertures of the head: two ears, two eyes, two nostrils, and the mouth.

63. SLEEP PEACEFULLY AND RECOVER AIR

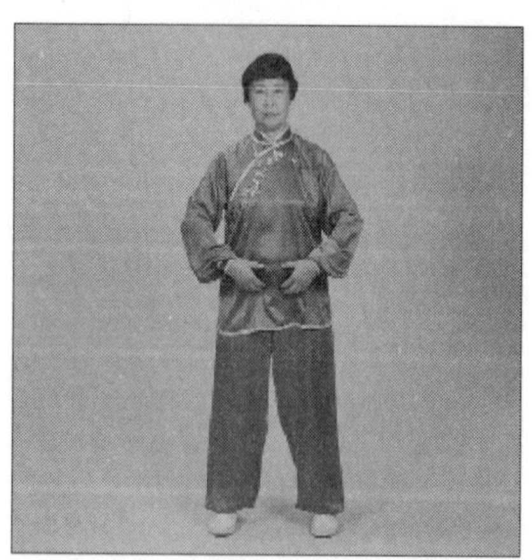

63 a-1. Bring the Shaking Palms down to the abdomen. Continue looking forward.

63 a-2. (CLOSE UP) Bring the Shaking Palms inward, and place them on the abdomen. When the Shaking Palms are placed on the abdomen, stop shaking, and slightly cup the palms (similar to the Scooping palm). The thumbs point towards each other, while the fingers point slightly towards each other. Keep the space between the thumb and forefinger open.

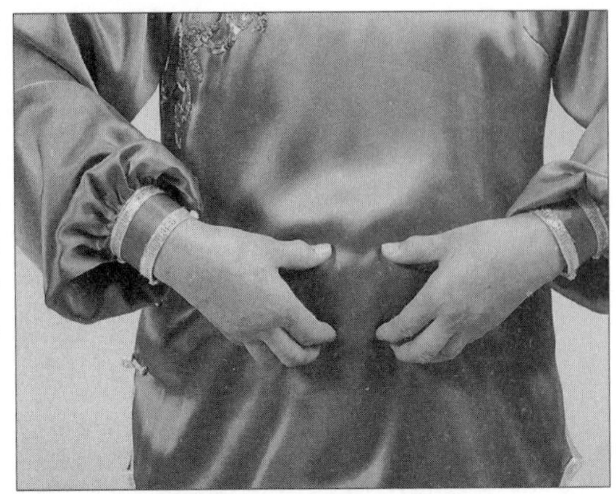

63 b-1. Keep the cupped palms on the abdomen. Gradually squat down on both legs, while gradually raising the heels upward. Let the head drop over, and relax.

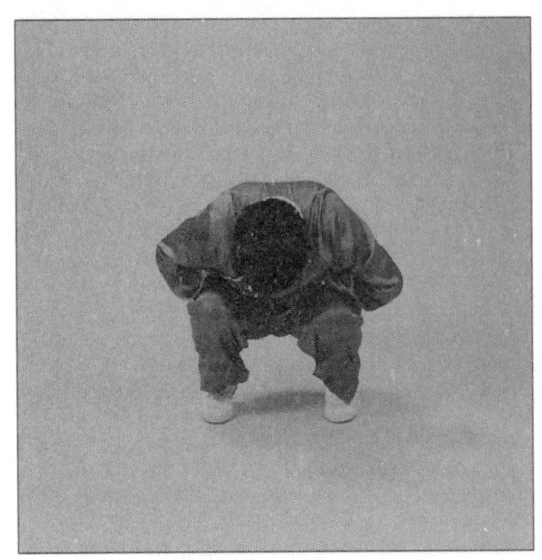

63 b-2. (ANOTHER ANGLE/CLOSE UP) The heels are raised off the ground, the buttocks tucked, the back is rounded and bent over, the head relaxes over, and the elbows rest on the knees; so the cupped hands can maintain contact with the abdomen. Relax for at least 30 seconds. Concentrate on the Lower Dantian. The eyes close, or are relaxed and half closed.

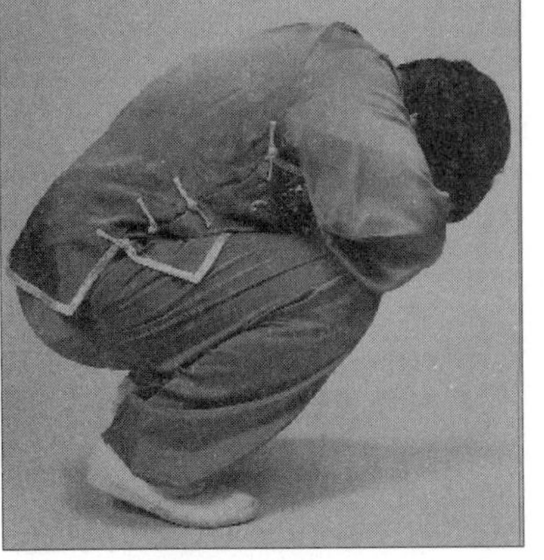

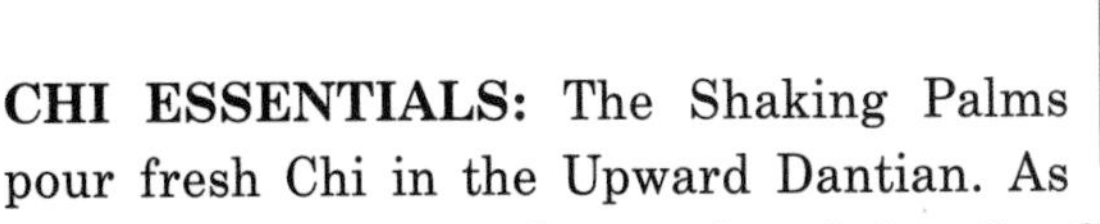

CHI ESSENTIALS: The Shaking Palms pour fresh Chi in the Upward Dantian. As the body squats into the two legs bring the Chi down. The cupped hands on the abdomen, the heels up, the tucked buttocks, the rounded back, and the head relaxed and hanging over focus all the body's intentions to bring the Chi down and store the Chi in the Lower Dantian for the purpose of strengthening the body's vital energy.

64. CLOSING POSITION (RECEIVE THE CHI)

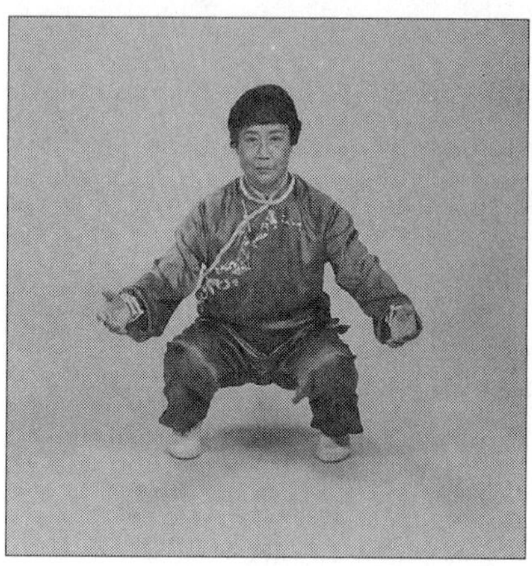

64 a. Open the eyes, look forward, and extend the hands forward. The palms face upward. Gradually stand up with the heels on the ground.

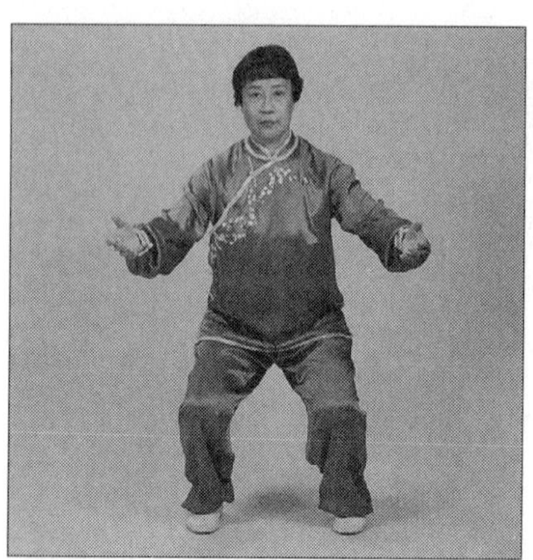

64 b. As the body gradually raises up, tuck the buttocks, and keep the torso erect. The eyes continue to look forward, and stand balanced.

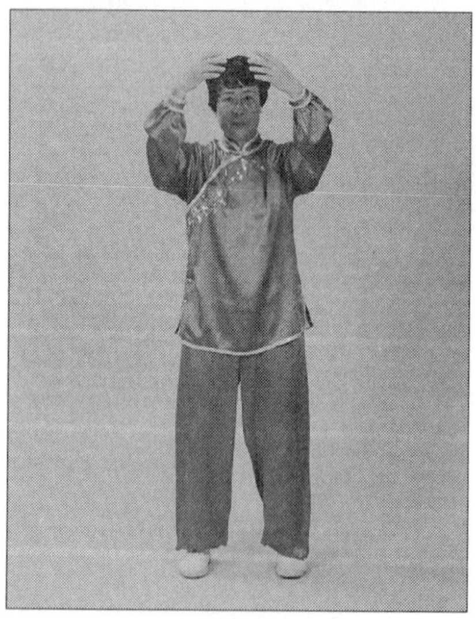

64 c. By the time you stand fully up, the palms raise up to forehead level. The palms face inward, so that the Laogong points on both palms face the Yintang point between the eyebrows.

64 d. Let the hands come down slowly and evenly paced. Hold no tightness in the joints, wrists, or upper limbs as the palms come down. Passing through the Shanzhong point (located between the nipples) and the Middle Dantian. Think of you arms sliding down an imaginary tree that the arms are embracing. The eyes look straight ahead.

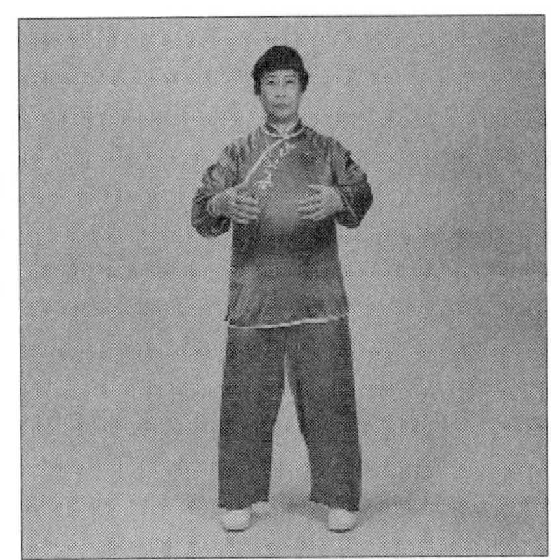

64 e. Let the palms gradually continue down to the Lower Dantian.

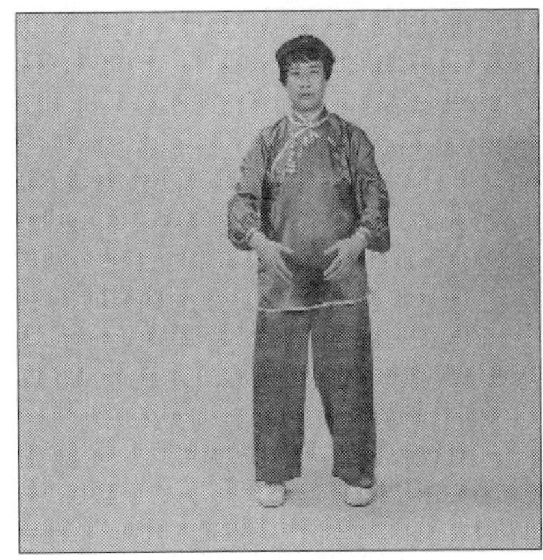

64 f. Bring the hands to the sides with the Chi sinking completely down into the Lower Dantian. Continue looking straight ahead.

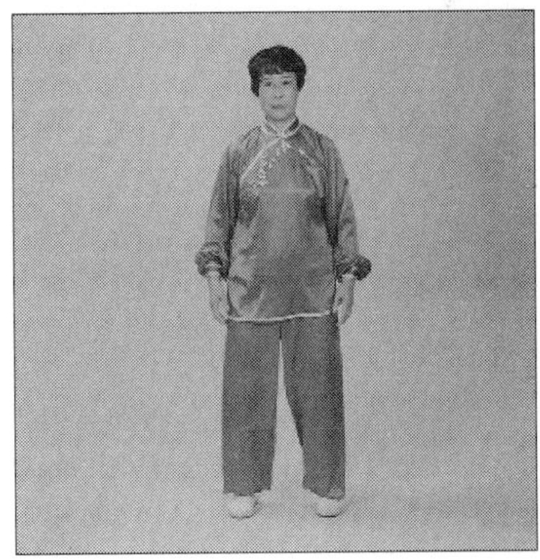

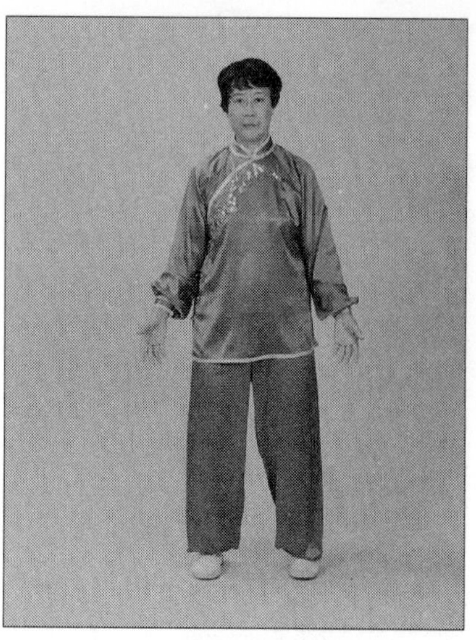

64 g. The palms turn outward, and then extend forward, outward, and upward.

Repeat movements 64 c through 64 g one more time, then do 64 c through 64 f, bringing the palms from Upward Dantian, through Middle Dantian, and to the Lower Dantian three times. Finally, do movement 64 h.

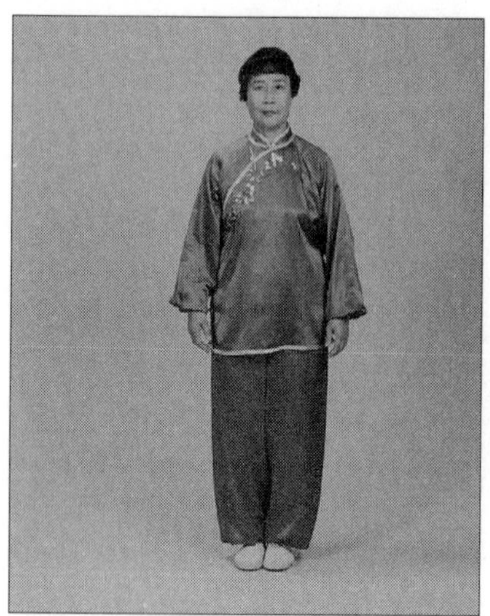

64 h. Softly and gently bring the left foot together with the right foot. Relax and stand very balanced. Look straight ahead into the distance.

CHI ESSENTIALS: It is essential to guide the Chi three times from Upward, Dantian through Middle Dantian, and to the Lower Dantian to receive and effectively store all the Chi developed from the entire form's practice.

CHAPTER EIGHT:

CONCLUSION

In conclusion, the authors wish to point out that this is only a brief look at the richness, depth, and diversity of the Wild Goose Chi Kung. They would like to receive information from experts in the field to improve the simple knowledge presented herein. Please overlook any mistakes, and realize that the authors are not perfect, and don't pretend to be. Wen Mei Yu and her student Gerald A. Sharp are still learning and in many ways beginners.

Presented herein is only a glimpse of the first 64 movements of a Chi Kung system which is one of the most popular of the oldest systems that exists in China today. In recent times, China has seen the development of great Chi Kung systems including the Guo Ling Chi Kung (also known as New Chi Kung) system and the Soaring Crane Chi Kung system. These systems are top notched and currently have many practitioners in China and throughout the world. It is fortunate to see any ancient system such as the Wild Goose Chi Kung system still remain as intact as it is today. However, systems such as the Taoist Five Thunder palm Chi Kung system of the Nine Dragon Wudang Mountain system, and the Wei Tuo (Shaolin Buddhist) system remain just a few of the ancient Chi Kung systems that remain intact and have top level practitioners sharing these rare arts with the public as well.

The authors hoped to have brought into the mainstream of Chi Kung practice ideas that will help shape and define ideas as to the path of the mystery known as Chi. In fact, they hope this book unravels the mystery of Chi, and that the knowledge shared in this book is useful to practitioners of martial arts (both external and internal), and persons from all walks of life.

It is intended that this book will shed light on the reality and practicality of Chi Kung, and how the practice of Chi Kung can be useful in everyday living. Hopefully, that people would spend as much time developing themselves through hard work and practice, as is spent on daily routines and tasks that make financial sense.

Finally, the authors wish that the art of Chi Kung will continue to be explored, researched, tested, and taught by great teachers and explored on a personal basis by those who dare to go inside themselves. Seeking to unravel the mystery that is "Chi" for themselves, and then to share with others their discoveries. All this in the name of an ancient Chinese healing art that continues to benefit all of humankind, and has done so now for thousands of years.

ABOUT THE AUTHOR

MASTER WEN MEI YU

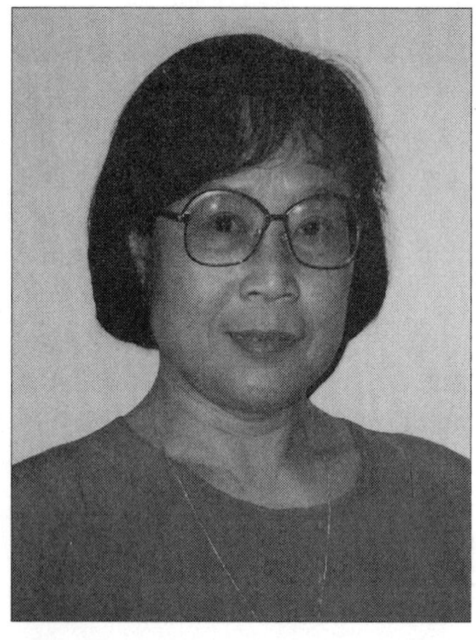

Born in 1936 in Shanghai, China, Wen Mei Yu was diagnosed with a bleeding ulcer at age 17. At that time Eastern, as well as Western medicine was ineffective. Her family and friends urged her to try Chi Kung (or, Qigong) practice.Reluctant, she tried to follow basic, simple methods of Chi Kung practice. In a very short time, she had great improvement in her health. Because of this she went on a journey into herself, and dedicated her life to the study of internal arts such as Taijiquan, Chi Kung, and related internal arts systems.

Wen Mei Yu learned Wild Goose (or, Dayan) Chi Kung directly from Yang Mei Jun, modern day exponent of the Taoist Kunlun School. In addition to Wild Goose Chi Kung, she studied several forms and systems of Chi Kung including: Contemporary forms such as: Guo Ling Chi Kung with Guo Ling, and Soaring Crane Chi Kung with Zhao Jin Xiang; and Traditional systems such as: Wei Tuo Chi Kung (Buddhist Shaolin), as well as the Wild Goose Chi Kung. Wen Mei Yu also had the great privilege to study in detail the Liangong Health Exercise system, developed by Dr. Zhuang Yuan Ming (a student of the legendary Wang Zhi Ping and Traditional Chinese Doctor of Traumatology).

Recipient of the All China Top Taijiquan Instructor Award in 1983, Wen Mei Yu is also highly noted for her practice of Taijiquan (Ta'i Chi Ch'uan). She studied the Wu style of Taijiquan and weapons with Wu Jian Quan's (Wu Chian Chuan) eldest daughter Wu Ying Hua, and Wu Jian Quan's son-in-law Ma Yueh Liang. She studied Yang style Taijiquan and weapons with Fu Zhong Wen (Yang Cheng Fu's nephew). She studied the Chen style with Gu Liu Xin (student of the legendary Chen Fake) whose books and material on the subject of Taijiquan continue to enlighten the public to this day. She also studied Chen style Taijiquan and contemporary forms of Taijiquan with Zhou Yuan Long whose drawings of Chen Fake, Chen Zhaokwei, Yang

Cheng Fu, Hao Shao Ru, Jiang Rong Qiao, Wu Jian Quan, and the 24 Simplified version of Taijiquan (To name only a few) continue to be used to this day for a variety books, periodicals, and publications. A great fan of Taijiquan, Wen Mei Yu is fond of Wu style Taijiquan and a senior member of the Chian Chuan TaiChiChuan Association, and has been a recognized active member and student since 1974.

Wen Mei Yu came to the United States in 1987 at the invitation of the International Kung Fu Federation. Not one to set on her laurels, Wen Mei Yu competed and won First Place in Hand Forms at the 2nd American Tai Chi Championships held in San Francisco in 1989, and First Place in Taiji Hands and Taiji Weapons Forms competitions at the World Cup held in Los Angeles in 1989.

She is the recipient of the "Award of Excellence" from the National Women's Martial Arts Federation. Internationally she has served as an instructor at the Women's Martial Arts Festival of Canada and for the Feminist International Summer Training Festival (also known as F.I.S.T.) held in the Netherlands and Europe. She has lectured and taught private lessons, group classes, and seminars throughout the United States and the world. She has taught people from various walks of life and abilities including: medical and health professionals, accident victims, cancer patients, persons with special needs (including disabilities), as well as other persons seeking personal development and enlightenment.

On a regular basis, Wen Mei Yu returns to China as often as she can to continue her studies in Taijiquan, Chi Kung, and related internal arts. Delving deeper into the tradition, as well as keeping up on contemporary research and developments in the internal arts. As a writer, she was recognized as Writer of the Year by *Inside Kung Fu* magazine.